the

grow

system

the
grow
system

The Essential Guide to
Modern Self-Sufficient Living—from
Growing Food to Making Medicine

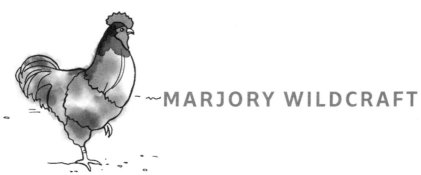

~MARJORY WILDCRAFT

AVERY an imprint of Penguin Random House New York

AVERY

an imprint of Penguin Random House LLC
penguinrandomhouse.com

Copyright © 2021 by Marjory Glowka
Illustrations by Alexis Seabrook
Penguin supports copyright. Copyright fuels creativity, encourages diverse voices, promotes free speech, and creates a vibrant culture. Thank you for buying an authorized edition of this book and for complying with copyright laws by not reproducing, scanning, or distributing any part of it in any form without permission. You are supporting writers and allowing Penguin to continue to publish books for every reader.

Most Avery books are available at special quantity discounts for bulk purchase for sales promotions, premiums, fund-raising, and educational needs. Special books or book excerpts also can be created to fit specific needs. For details, write SpecialMarkets @penguinrandomhouse.com.

Library of Congress Cataloging-in-Publication Data

Names: Wildcraft, Marjory, author.
Title: The grow system: true health, wealth, and happiness come from the ground / Marjory Wildcraft.
Description: New York: Avery, an imprint of Penguin Random House LLC, [2021] | Includes index.
Identifiers: LCCN 2020057426 (print) | LCCN 2020057427 (ebook) | ISBN 9780593330364 (paperback) | ISBN 9780593330371 (ebook)
Subjects: LCSH: Gardening—Therapeutic use. | Medicinal plants. | Alternative medicine.
Classification: LCC RM735.7.G37 W53 2021 (print) | LCC RM735.7.G37 (ebook) | DDC 615.8/515—dc23
LC record available at https://lccn.loc.gov/2020057426
LC ebook record available at https://lccn.loc.gov/2020057427

p.   cm.

Printed in the United States of America
2nd Printing

Book design by Lorie Pagnozzi

This book is dedicated to Earth, the heavens, the plants, and all the creatures. And to you. Hopefully, from reading this book you begin to get a glimmer into the truth of the reality that we are all One.

contents

part III
safeguard your family, now and for the future

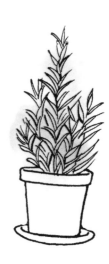

introduction

I have always been interested in wealth. I grew up in a family who sort of hovered above the poverty line, and like most people, I thought "wealth" meant accumulating a big pile of money. After my first career as an electrical engineer and consultant, I studied with Robert Kiyosaki (of *Rich Dad Poor Dad* fame) and launched my own real estate investment business. I did well and amassed a portfolio of 65 houses I was leasing to tenants with an option to buy. I had built a successful career and was earning a good income for me and my family.

Even though the business was doing well, my intuition kept telling me something was wrong. Being successful in real estate meant carrying a lot of debt, and Fannie Mae and Freddie Mac were essentially my biggest partners. I began to study their business models and soon realized they contained some fundamental problems that made me worry about what would happen should an economic downtown occur. If the tenants could no longer afford rent, my investors and I could easily get stuck with a lot of highly leveraged properties and no income to pay them off—a terrifying prospect that kept me up at night. Essentially foreseeing the financial crash of 2008, I decided to unwind my investments. Although some of my investors initially were upset that I was going to shut down the portfolio when everything seemed fine, eventually every single one of them thanked me profusely.

I understood that we were about to enter a period that would be extremely difficult and affect everyone. Throughout human history, humans have faced challenges and changes that involve tremendous upheaval and hardship: natural disasters, civil wars, hyperinflation, totalitarian regimes, plagues, and pandemics. The recent COVID-19 global pandemic has shown us how quickly these changes can happen, from lack of access to medical care and unemployment to empty grocery store shelves. On some gut level, we understand that our supply chains—and our entire way of life—are extremely vulnerable.

I wanted to learn everything I could about how people had survived such crises in the past and what I'd need most for my family's safety and well-being. Security and medical access are big issues, but while doing historical research and interviews I saw over and over again that the most difficult part of navigating a tumultuous period is consistent access to food.

Around the same time, I led a project at a nearby elementary school to provide locally grown food to students as a healthier lunch option and to also teach them about the health and environmental benefits of eating local fruits and vegetables. The project seemed like a slam dunk because just about everyone was behind it—the parents, the school administration, the community, and even the kids, who started a small schoolyard garden and loved tending to it. Grant money, at both federal and state levels, also was available. I saw it as a trial project we could eventually roll out to the entire state. We project leaders knew nearly all the farmers who were growing organically in Texas and enthusiastically began making a list of all the farmers who could provide the food for the project.

That's when we realized there weren't enough local farmers in the county, or even the surrounding counties, to provide all the vegetables for this one small rural elementary school. I had always thought there was food in the countryside, but I soon learned the harsh truth: the small farm network has been completely dismantled. Let me repeat that. In the entire county—and Texas has some big counties—there were not enough vegetables being grown to make part of the lunches for one small rural elementary school. The horror of this slammed through me.

Sometimes the universe needs to send you a crisis to open you to a new perspective. After learning how little food was available locally, I was terrified by the enormity of what could happen to my family and my community. I couldn't sleep and felt panicked. In my despair, I came to one simple and humble conclusion: I would have to grow food.

I do not come from a farming background, nor was my family the "live off the land" type, so I set out to learn everything I could about how to grow food. I started with my own garden and several of my favorite vegetables. After a while, I added a few animals I could raise on my own. Pretty soon I became interested in herbal medicine and how it might help me—both my health and my pocketbook. I spent hours studying gardening books and watching instructional videos to develop my skills. I knew I wanted to produce deeply nutritious, organic, clean food in a truly sustainable way so I'd always know I could feed my family.

I've made some mistakes, but I take pride in the skills I've developed. My family and I grow nearly all our food—enough to feed a family of four—and support our farm with only a small portion of store-bought feed for our animals. I feel a deep sense of security when I look out the back door at our yard full of edible, useful, and medicinal plants and animals and in our pantry, where every shelf is laden with jars of fruit, vegetables, and meat we've canned.

Ultimately, I discovered the powerful solution I had been searching for, but I also realized something even more important. At one point in my life, I was excited about moving up the corporate ladder and potentially becoming vice president of a multinational company. In my real estate career, I was thrilled to broker bigger and bigger deals to give my investors huge returns. Now I know that the simple act of growing your own food—and the love and sense of community that work brings to your life—is so much more rewarding. It is the source of true wealth. And perhaps the biggest satisfaction of all is the incredible bonding that has developed among my family as we have worked together to grow our food, tend to our farm, and help treat common illnesses with homemade remedies.

The Grow Network

As my family and I continued to see success from our efforts, I decided to share my knowledge with like-minded others. I put together a workshop for my neighbors and community members to teach them how they, too, could make better use of their own backyards. My workshops were so popular, I got calls to turn them into a video that could reach others outside my community. I filmed a video that would become my *Grow Your Own Groceries* DVD, created a website to support and build community around it in 2009, and The Grow Network was born.

The Grow Network has become an international community of hundreds of thousands of members and provides resources for many more. My followers have learned how satisfying it is to take care of themselves and their family—without having to go to a doctor for every little ailment, without relying only on prescription medications, and without having to accept what's available at their local grocery stores as the only option to feed their family.

I'm not advocating that people live completely off the grid, unless that's what they want. I get my bloodwork checked every year by a doctor. I buy things in stores when I want to. But I also know that the bulk of my and my family's needs can be met in my own backyard. It's a truly empowering and purposeful way of life.

About This Book

This way of life is also completely doable, and that's where *The Grow System* comes in. Starting The Grow Network has shown me that I'm not the only one who wants to live like this—far from it. It's also shown me that most people don't think it's possible to achieve. They think they don't have the time or the space or the ability. But they couldn't be more wrong!

In this book I show you how to set up the three-part Grow System so you can successfully grow half the food you need in your own backyard by working at it less than an hour a day. I also teach you how to treat the 12 most common ailments you and your family members are likely to encounter—without relying on the pharmaceutical industry or going to a doctor.

These are the fundamental skills I introduce in this book, but *The Grow System* offers so much more. It gives you the tools you need to live a healthier, more sustainable, more self-sufficient life. It can be used as a starting point for beginners who have no experience whatsoever with plants, animals, or herbs. It is also meant to be a valuable resource for those who have some experience with gardening or home medicine and are ready to elevate their skills in a systematic way to build true wealth and independence and really improve their or others' lives. Throughout the book I share plenty of anecdotes about my family's experience starting our farm and growing our own food to illustrate how easily it can be done.

Not very long ago, practically everyone was living this way. Your grandmother probably had a kitchen garden, and she almost certainly did not have a CVS to run to when someone in the family got sick. These skills are more important than ever. We may have lost some of the knowledge, but we're still capable of all the things our ancestors used to do as part of their everyday lives. It's time to rediscover their secrets and create a stronger connection to the powerful force of nature. In fact, it's urgent that we do. When we get back in touch with that self-sufficient spirit, we are safer and our lives are so much richer because of it.

Consider this advice from Saint Francis of Assisi: "Start by doing what's necessary, then do what's possible, and suddenly you are doing the impossible."

Read on, and I'll show you how to take that next step.

the
grow
system

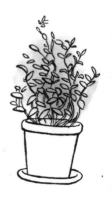

grow
your own
groceries

chapter 1

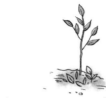

true wealth comes from the **ground**

I can't do that."

That was the knee-jerk reaction of my friend Maria, whom I knew when I was living in Austin, Texas, as I told her I'd gotten into producing my own food and medicine. She looked at me as if I was doing the impossible. It wasn't that she wasn't interested. "I'd love to be able to do what you do," she told me. "I just don't think I could."

I understood where she was coming from. She was a busy urban professional with a husband and young children to take care of. She didn't think she had the time. She wasn't sure she had enough room in her city backyard. She had no experience gardening or raising animals. Plus, she didn't cook a lot of meals with fresh ingredients and relied a lot on packaged food (and the occasional takeout dinner) to feed her family. How could she possibly take on such a time-consuming project?

After listening to all her self-defeating talk, I made a suggestion. "Look, Maria, you don't have to do everything I'm doing. Why don't you start with just a few herbs on your windowsill and see where it takes you?"

I recommended she start with some of the easiest-to-grow herbs, like basil, oregano, chives, or thyme. These are very hardy—and hard-to-kill—plants. Plus, they are fundamental and delicious ingredients to use when cooking.

For each herb, I suggested she get the biggest pot that would fit on her windowsill. The bigger the pot, the more soil and water it could hold. This would help her herbs if she wasn't exactly consistent with her watering schedule at first. They would still thrive until she developed the habit of checking them every day.

Finally, I advised she put the herbs in a place she visited frequently. On a sunny windowsill over the kitchen sink is often the best place because most people are near their sink each day on a regular basis and would remember to care for the plants more often. Tucking them away in a spare bedroom or another area that doesn't get much traffic could mean they'd be forgotten.

Maria followed my advice. She started growing a handful of different herbs and then began using them in her everyday recipes. She put fresh basil on pasta, added fresh rosemary to her weekly chicken dish, and garnished soups with chopped fresh chives.

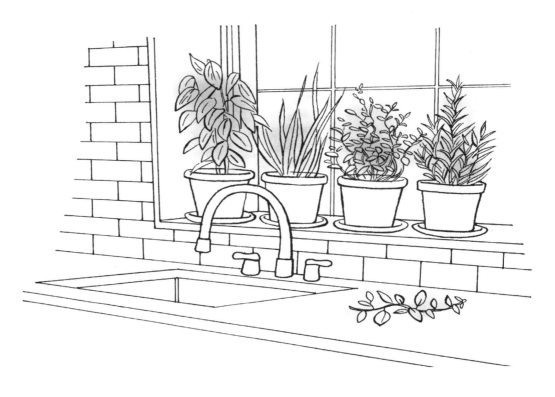

It is astonishing what a difference adding fresh herbs makes to the flavor of a dish. Maria not only enjoyed the meals more herself, but she also knew something magical was happening when her husband started asking her if she was cooking with new recipes. (The recipes weren't new; the only difference was the bit of fresh herbs.) Most satisfying to Maria was that her kids began asking for seconds and talking about how good their mom's cooking was.

The fresh herbs had such a positive effect on their nightly dinner routine that Maria decided to try something more. She set aside a few square feet in her backyard to grow squash and tomatoes. Then she added a few more square feet for some greens. It snowballed from there, and pretty soon she added some chickens and then some rabbits.

Along the way, she started noticing some changes she hadn't expected.

Because they were enjoying her food so much, her family got involved and helped her tend the garden. Maria's kids especially loved helping pick that evening's fresh food, and soon it became something they all worked on together.

Maria also saw changes in her health. After about a year of eating out of her own backyard, she realized the nightmarish allergies she'd always suffered from had disappeared.

These positive benefits sparked her interest in herbal medicine, and soon another new world opened for her.

Maria still had her career and her busy family life, but she now viewed her life with renewed purpose. When Maria first became a mom, she felt strongly that caring for her family was her most important and rewarding job. But somehow it still felt somewhat empty, like she was just part of a processing line packed with conveniences. She felt like a cog in the "buy food, microwave it, and serve it to the kids" machine. She didn't think she had time to cook with fresh ingredients, even though the health of her family was extremely important to her. But by learning a few new skills and turning her backyard into a "grow system," Maria began to tap into the power to deeply nourish and heal those around her. In that ability to create, she found the joy and fulfillment she had hoped for in becoming a mother.

The Five Keys to True Wealth

I am an extremely wealthy woman. And after all she's learned, Maria would say the same about herself.

Now, do either of us have a vacation house in Aspen or a penthouse in New York? No. Do we drive fancy cars? Not unless you consider an old pickup truck "fancy." We both have some money in the bank but no extensive portfolio of stocks or bonds.

Right now, you may be asking yourself how Maria and I can call ourselves wealthy. But in my mind, it's time we looked at the idea of "wealth" in a different way. We live in strange times, full of rapid change and lots of uncertainty. We need to crawl out of the dark, narrow chasm that defines "wealth" only as financial assets. True wealth is about a lot more than money. It's about the things we have that make life worth living! As I see it, to truly be wealthy, you need five basic things:

1. Health
2. Family
3. Community
4. Meaningful work
5. Purpose

These five things are what make a rich life.

After all, what good is a big bank account if you are in pain, have no energy, and don't enjoy living in your own body? What good is a nice house if you don't have strong and loving relationships with your family and can't share it with them? What's the meaning of a fancy job title if you don't have a fulfilling purpose in your life? What joy is there if you don't have friends to share in life's adventures? There is nothing emptier and more demeaning than working just for money. You are here for a reason that goes beyond your financial destiny, and your life energy is too precious to waste on anything that does not make a deep and lasting contribution to yourself and to others. Most of us know in our hearts that money is not what makes us feel happy and whole.

Have you gone to your high school reunions through the years? I've found it quite fascinating to see the focus of various times. In your twenties and thirties, for example, everyone was eyeing the attractiveness of your spouse, how much money you were bringing in, or what splashes you had made in the media. As the years and decades roll by, the focus shifts to who is the healthiest and most independent of the medical system. Health, family, community, meaningful work, and purpose are the things that make our lives full and satisfying. You don't need to go to graduate school, slave away at a desk, or get a job on Wall Street to become truly wealthy. In fact, you are unlikely to find real wealth in those places at all.

You can find everything you need to create immense amounts of true wealth in your own backyard. Specifically, you can cultivate all five aspects of wealth by learning to do two basic things: grow your own food and make your own medicine.

Gardening, raising chickens, and practicing herbal medicine are becoming increasingly popular in rural and urban America alike, but what I want to propose in this book is that they are so much more than hobbies. They are the foundation upon which any one of us can build a healthy, satisfying, empowering, and truly wealthy life.

Finding Your Way

In Part I of the book, I explain how to grow food in your backyard. I also show you that it is not only a fun and satisfying pastime but also something that will increase your wealth in a whole host of ways:

 Food you produce yourself is more nutritious than grocery store offerings, and you can choose growing methods that align with your values—natural, organic, pesticide-free, pasture-raised (your backyard certainly counts as "local"). Actually, the *process* of growing food is more **health-giving** than simply eating nutritious ingredients. You will be spending time in the sun, connecting with nature, and engaging in gentle movements and stretches—all good for your overall well-being.

Growing, gathering, preparing, and eating food together has been the primary glue that has held **families** together throughout history. Harvesting and cooking with your kids, collaborating on dishes with your spouse, and sharing food at family gatherings creates memories and builds strong family ties that last.

Gifting, exchanging, bartering, and trading products from your backyard production builds **community** at a basic level. You can work together with your neighbors to grow calorie crops, raise animals, go on foraging trips, harvest, and process bounties, fostering deep relationships as you do so.

There is no more **meaningful work** than creating highly nutritious, deeply healing foods for your loved ones, while healing the bit of Earth that exists in your backyard at the same time. Of course, this also has benefits for a more traditional notion of work (that is, making money) by saving on the high costs of buying healthy, organic, local food.

Your work in your backyard is deeply **purposeful**. Becoming more self-reliant is empowering, living more harmoniously with the natural environment helps restore our beautiful planet, and you can create a legacy developing your own varieties of seeds or breeds of livestock that future generations will be grateful to you for.

Part II of this book teaches you how to use local plants and herbs to naturally and gently treat a host of common medical issues you and your family are likely to experience. As with food production, this knowledge and ability will increase your wealth in the same five important ways:

Knowing how to make and use your own remedies for common ailments, like colds or burns, builds **health**, as does the deep nutrition available through herbal infusions. These options are generally safer and more effective than what can be found at the drugstore and are welcome options for those with concerns about the toxicities in drugs and supplements.

Becoming the primary health-care giver in your **family** is a role that builds bonds, trust, and love at a deep level with family members. I love that my grown children still ask me for elderberry cough syrup or fire cider to help them through the winter, and they've seen me through maladies as well, including a snakebite!

Trading, sharing, and swapping medicines and herbs within your extended circle builds **community** far better than any Tupperware party can. Helping neighbors through illness and swapping stories of what has worked creates deeper relationships.

There is no more **meaningful work** than making medicines that contribute to the healing of your family and friends and help them feel better. As with producing your own food, making your own medicines can save you money, considering the high costs of pharmaceutical and natural treatments.

Starting a family "herbal book," in which you record who got sick and how the illness was treated, creates a family record that may sentimentally surpass the family Bible or photo album. An herbal book tells a highly personal and **purposeful** story of your family history and passes on the family healing knowledge to future generations.

Having this kind of wealth easily accessible when you walk out your own back door—or even just on your windowsills like Maria had when she started—can really change your life for the better, and it's a lot more doable than you think. This book shows you how, step by step, and gives you all the tools you need to become a billionaire in true wealth.

chapter summary

- You don't have to do it all at once. Small changes can bring big improvements.

- True wealth is about making your life worth living.

- The five keys to wealth are health, family, community, meaningful work, and purpose.

- You can find everything you need to create immense amounts of true wealth in your own backyard.

- You can cultivate all five aspects of wealth by learning to grow your own food and make your own medicine.

additional resources

For more information on getting started with gardening, check out these websites:

- www.TrueWealthQuiz.com. A fun assessment tool to determine your level of true wealth.

- www.AlandFood.com. A fascinating interview with Dr. Kai-Fu Lee, the world's leading expert on artificial intelligence (AI). Dr. Lee discusses how AI will help or hinder backyard food production, how it will affect commercial agribusiness, and AI's impact on our society in general.

- www.YourPlaceOnEarth.com. A few short questions you can use to discover which of the nine regions on Earth you live in. You'll find out what grows best where you live, learn what medicines are easiest to find there, and connect with other people who live in your region.

chapter 2

the garden:
growing your own food is like
printing your own money

I was nervous. Although I had excitedly volunteered to teach gardening at a local school, now I was in front of a group of uninterested middle-schoolers, and I was seriously wondering how big this failure would be. Very few of these children ate vegetables regularly, cheap fast food was a staple, and most of them were envious when another student showed up with a Lunchable in their pack.

I did have some things working in my favor to get their attention. Being outside on the sunny playground was definitely a step up from being inside the classroom. The kids were happy to do practical work and help construct the raised bed garden. Showing them how to safely use the power drill to screw the boards together conveyed trust and built confidence. And even though some of the kids were a little small, they took on the challenge of using the grown-up shovels to unload the truck and fill the bed. They loved the rich smell and moist, crumbly feel of the dark earth between their fingers as they shaped and smoothed the soil.

I beamed at how excited and tender they were while transplanting the starts and taking on the duties of regular watering and weeding. I had chosen some strawberries and snap peas to plant—classic favorites that are pretty much guaranteed to go over well with kids, but in most of the garden, I had them plant oak leaf lettuce, kale, turnips, chard, radishes, mustard greens, and broccoli.

That was what made me worried. The only salad many of these kids had ever eaten was wilted iceberg lettuce and perhaps a pale, sad excuse for a tomato. They had never tasted most of what we were growing. If I could get them to try the kale, would they spit it out?

A few weeks later, when the greens got big enough to start picking (they come up pretty quickly), I put some small containers of ranch dressing in the classroom fridge. I showed the kids how to harvest a lettuce leaf, dip it in the dressing, and eat it, and I let them know they could do that whenever they wanted.

When eating the greens started to become a "thing" at recess, I was fist pumping and jumping with joy. The kids absolutely loved the lettuce, kale, chard, and broccoli. The spicy zing of the mustard greens and radishes was an exciting flavor most had never experienced before, and they ate it up. After a while, the children didn't even need the ranch dressing to enjoy the veggies. They started munching on the greens directly from the garden between games of tag or hide-and-seek.

My advice to those of you who say you don't like vegetables is . . . try homegrown. If you've never eaten homegrown vegetables, then you've never really eaten vegetables! The vegetables you find at your supermarket are grown using industrial methods that give them a bland flavor. They also have to make a multiple-day journey through the supply chain between when they are picked and arrive at your market. Homegrown produce is almost like a different food group. Its bright taste and freshness are unmatched, and it can win over even the pickiest eaters.

My own kids were raised on homegrown food, and growing up, they loved vegetables. But on the rare occasion when I purchased store-bought broccoli, it would be left on the dinner table untouched, alone, and uneaten. Good produce has always been part of my family's lives, and they have developed discerning palates.

More Than Just a Garden

I probably don't have to tell you that if you opt to buy pesticide-free, organic produce—foods that are healthier for both you and the environment—you are looking at some high grocery bills. But when you grow your own tomatoes and other favorite foods, you'll be amazed by how much money you can save.

Along with the cost-saving benefits, having easy access to fresh vegetables from your backyard will transform your meals and dramatically improve your family's habits and health. A backyard garden also helps strengthen your relationship with your community.

I really felt the power of my strongly knit community a number of years ago when I got a call from a guy I knew who had recently started an organic greenhouse to grow tomatoes. His first attempt at growing them had failed, and so did his second, but the third time was a charm. He produced so many tomatoes, he didn't know what to do with them all.

"Hey, Marjory," he said to me when I answered the phone. "If I showed up tomorrow with a trailerful of fresh, organic, fully ripe tomatoes, would you want them?"

"Give me five minutes to figure it out, and I'll get back to you," I told him. I then called two neighbors, and within minutes, we had organized a community canning party at one of their homes. The next day, my entire family and several others showed up to slice and dice tomatoes, sterilize the jars, and pack them full. The kids were there, occasionally helping out and occasionally running out. One neighbor had an eight-month-old, and whoever needed a break would take a turn holding the baby. It was a magical, wonderful day filled with good food, great company, and lots of useful work. At the end of it, each family went home with two years' worth of fresh, delicious tomato sauce.

Now in our community, when one of us has a bumper crop of something, we share it. If we need help with a big harvest, we call the neighbors. We've formed an incredible support system, and all our lives are richer, more fun, and more secure as a result.

I want to create a movement of families and communities who have these kinds of strong bonds, better health, greater happiness, and more self-sufficiency. I want people to come together to increase the value and meaning in their own lives. But we've got to take the first steps to make that happen! An oak doesn't spring up from the ground fully grown. You have to start small, with practical, manageable goals.

So how do you get started? In the following section, I give you step-by-step instructions with a basic "recipe" for creating your own backyard garden. Then I offer tips for taking it to the next level and provide inspiration to keep you going.

The Basic Recipe for Your Backyard Garden

Before I dive into this garden recipe, my biggest piece of advice is that you start small. You really don't need a huge garden to produce the amount of vegetables your family will really need—it's amazing what a small garden can produce. You'll also be much more successful if you begin with a size you can manage.

Start with a 50- or 100-square-foot garden at most. When I worked with the schoolkids, we created a 50-square-foot garden bed. I planted many "cut and come again" greens like kale, spinach, and lettuces, which means you can harvest the leaves and come back again and again. The garden produced plenty of greens for 13 grazing kids for four months! I talk more about exactly what and how to plant later in this chapter, but the big message for now is to start slowly and then grow (pun intended!) from there.

To start your garden you'll need the following:

Ingredients
Sunlight
Raised beds
Soil
Water
Seeds and/or starts

Sunlight

Choose a sunny spot for your garden because sunlight is one of the foods your plants require. Most vegetables need at least 6 hours of direct sunlight to produce, and more is better. If you are not sure what kind of sun an area in your backyard gets, pick a day; take six to eight photos throughout the day in the morning, afternoon, and evening; and record what you see. (Now is a great time to start your garden journal! More on that coming up.)

You also want to choose a spot near a back or kitchen door because the closer your garden is to your house, the more you'll pay attention to and use it. This is why our grandparents used to have what they called "kitchen gardens."

Again, you want to start small! A 50-square-foot (4×12.5-feet) bed is a perfect beginner size. You won't need much more than that for now. Eventually you can work up to a total of 100 square feet, or two 50-square-foot beds, if you want to grow more. In terms of dimensions, create beds that are between 4 and a maximum of 5 feet wide so you'll be able to reach to the center easily.

Here is a drawing of what 100 square feet of garden made from two 50-square-foot raised beds looks like.

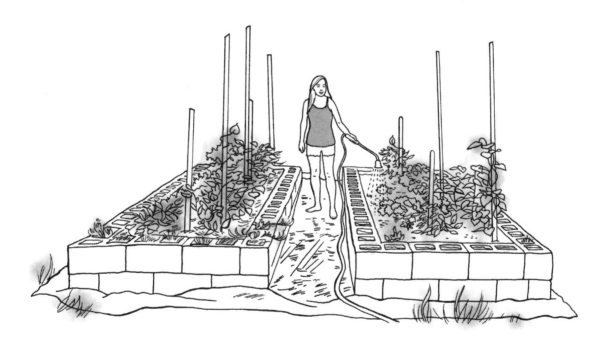

Raised Beds

I recommend starting out with raised beds. Soil is what gives vegetables their nutrition and flavor, and unfortunately, most of us have poor native soils in our backyards. Using raised beds is an easy way to solve this problem and begin your garden with high-quality growing soil.

Raised beds are quick, easy, and inexpensive to construct, and you have some choices when it comes to building material.

Cinder Blocks

I like to use cinder blocks because they are inexpensive, durable, and only weigh about 16 pounds each, so they are not hard to move (even for children!). You don't need to mortar or glue the blocks together as you build your beds because they will stay in place if set well. I used to work with military families who moved every two years to a new base. It wasn't the lightest move ever, but when it came time to move, they bagged up their soil, stacked up their cinder blocks, and transported their gardens to their new homes.

Wood

The next most common material used to make raised beds is wooden boards. If you go with wood, I recommend either 2×8- or 2×12-inch planks stacked two high so the border is 16 or 24 inches tall. Pine is the least expensive and most widely available, and it's a good option. Cedar will last much longer than pine and is also fine to use. For many years, using pressure-treated wood was not recommended for raised bed gardens because it was produced with a compound that contained arsenic, but apparently the lumber industry has changed and no longer uses that compound. There is still some debate about it (of course), but the newer pressure-treated wood intended for ground contact landscaping is now considered safe; does not contain leachable arsenic; and lasts many, many more years than untreated lumber.

Other Options

You don't have to use wood or cinder blocks, you can get creative and think outside the box! I've seen beds made out of old horse watering troughs and others created from recycled roofing sheet metal for the sides and T-posts for the supports. Even old bathtubs can work—they have sloped drainage (although, ideally, it's better to have a few holes in the bottom for drainage). My friend Abi grew greens in the open cavity of an old grand piano!

A while back I was involved in a huge debate over the safety of growing food in old tires. You can make a quick small raised bed by cutting out the sidewalls of tires and stacking up cylindrical shells. The question was, Will the tires leach out noxious stuff that your plants will take up? The debate is still raging on. I decided that for my beds, I'd turn the tires inside out so the tread side is on the inside surface. My thinking is that after so many miles of use, the tread has been exposed to rain, air, wear, and tear and has probably released most of its objectionable toxins.

Constructing Your Bed

Regardless of what material you decide to use, a depth of 16 to 24 inches with good drainage is ideal for a raised bed. Before you begin construction, clear the ground both underneath the bed and a perimeter of at least 18 inches around the sides of the bed. Grass and weeds have an astonishing desire to grow. Many people incorrectly think 2 feet of soil is enough to suppress the grass and weeds, but they will grow right up through that soil and thank you for providing such a wonderful habitat. Another common mistake is that people forget to clear a good border around the beds that is completely free of grass. Just because you create a boundary by putting up a board does not mean the grass won't cross it.

I also recommend that you line the bottom of your raised beds and your surrounding perimeter with a heavy-duty landscaping cloth, which will help continue to suppress any remaining and emerging grass competition. The cloth should be permeable to water so it drains and won't get waterlogged. If you use that old horse trough, make lots of good drainage holes in the bottom and then line it with gravel.

And one last note: please don't think I'm "antigrass." I love grasses! There is a wonderful saying that all flesh is grass, and if you spend some time thinking about that, you'll find it's true. But grasses often out-compete the garden vegetables you are trying to grow and will cause your production to be low or even nonexistent.

Soil

You can build up your own soil over a period of years, but starting off with good, living, nutrient-rich soil will give you a big head start and increase your probability of success. Really great soil helps control pests and insects, reduces watering needs, and makes your garden so much easier to take care of.

How much soil do you need? A 50-square-foot garden made from cinder blocks is approximately 16 inches deep and requires a volume of 67 cubic feet, or about 2.5 cubic yards of soil. Here's what that amount looks like in practical terms:

- A 40-pound bag of soil is 0.75 cubic feet, or 0.03 cubic yards. You need 90 bags.

- A large wheelbarrow holds about a tenth of a cubic yard of soil. You need 25 wheelbarrows full.

- A midsize Ford F-150 pickup truck bed is approximately 2.3 cubic yards. You need a heaping truckload.

The definitions of "garden soil," "topsoil," and "landscaping soil" are very loose, and the quality of these types of soil can vary widely. Look for soil that is dark, crumbly, moist, and smells earthy.

The best place to get quality soil is from a local organic nursery owned by a proprietor who knows how and where the soil was created. The next best thing is to call some local landscaping contractors and ask them for the best-quality soil they can find. Try to get a sample of it first if you can. Asking around at a local garden club is another great way of finding good sources of soil and compost.

If you can't find, or just can't afford, high-quality soil, do the best you can with what you have. You can add high-quality compost, minerals, and soil microbes to your existing soil to improve its quality and nutrients.

It's important to keep in mind that even if you start out with great soil, to keep the soil healthy and happy, you need to add compost and fertilizers regularly. (I talk about this a lot more in Chapter 5.)

bio sludge

I applaud the many municipalities that are composting solid wastes, but when it comes to soils or composts for your garden, definitely stay away from this stuff. Known as "bio sludge" among gardeners, it is just what you are thinking—the composted wastes from everything everyone flushes down the public sewage system. It is loaded with heavy metals, cleaning chemicals, pharmaceuticals, and an array of things you do not want in your yard, much less your garden.

Unfortunately, bio sludge is being used as a fertilizer in some commercial agriculture food crops, which is yet another reason to grow your own. As of this writing, its use is prohibited for production in anything that is certi-fied USDA organic, but it is still used as an ingredient in various nonorganic bagged compost and soil mixtures sold in stores. In the Austin, Texas, area, one of the brands of soils made with bio sludge is called Dillo Dirt; in Seattle, Washington, there's GroCo. Some are clearly labeled "not for use in produc-ing food crops," but some are not. Definitely read the package and avoid anything that lists "bio solids" or "activated sewage" in the ingredients.

Water

Be sure to set up a watering system for your garden *before* you plant. Even if you live in a part of the country where there's usually enough rainfall, most places have a dry season or periods when you will need to supplement rain with watering.

A very rough guideline is that a garden needs a total of about 1 inch of water per week. Obviously, you'll need more water in the high desert and much less in the wet tropics, and your schedule will be different depending on your region. In the high desert, you'll water almost daily, and in the wet tropics, you'll water only occasionally.

I highly recommend hand-watering with a hose and a good wand attachment (it's part of the secret to a green thumb I talk about later in this chapter), but feel free to set up a sprinkler on a timer for consistent watering when you aren't home to do it.

Also, it's important to remember that when you are watering, you are watering the *soil*, not the plants, so have your wand down closer to the roots.

Here are some more tips on the best sources for water:

> Rainwater. The best water to use for your garden is rainwater. It's magical how a garden will perk up after a good rain. It's the gold standard. But rain doesn't come on schedule in most places, so collecting it and saving it is necessary for consistent watering pretty much everywhere. For a 50-square-foot garden, 1 inch of rain is approximately 31 gallons of water. In many areas of the country, a 55-gallon drum collecting rain off the roof is sufficient to water a 50-square-foot bed.

> Pond water. After rainwater, one of the next-best sources of water is pond water, especially if it has fish in it because the fish poop adds a natural fertilizer to the water.

> Well water. Well water is often another good source of water, assuming you've tested it for various toxins such as pesticides, herbicides, or petroleum-type contaminants, which are surprisingly (and disturbingly) common.

> Municipal water. Municipal water is often the least-desirable water because it contains either chlorine or chloramine. But if that's all you have, do the best you can with it. Your city or town should have a readily available report on how your water is treated. If your water contains chlorine, let it sit uncovered (perhaps in a 55-gallon drum) for 24 hours or so to let the chlorine evaporate. Chloramine, which is more common in municipal water supplies, won't evaporate. But both chlorine and chloramine can be bound up by humates, which are found in good, aged compost. You also can buy a bottle of liquid humates at any gardening store. About 1 cup of humates to 50 gallons of municipal water is sufficient in most places—it all depends on how much your municipality concentrates the chemicals. Another simple strategy is to spread a good layer of compost and mulch as the top layer (almost like a sacrifice layer) in your garden bed. It will act like a filter to deactivate the chloramine.

Plantings

To get my garden started, I do a combination of transplanting starts and direct seeding. I suggest you do both, too.

Starts

In many places, the outdoor growing season just isn't long enough for a seed planted directly into the ground to have enough time to grow into a plant and produce a vegetable, so many gardeners start seeds indoors in small trays in the late winter to give their plants a head start.

Starts also are more space- and time-efficient to grow in trays or small pots indoors and then transplant out into the big garden when they are a few inches high and ready. Your garden can be producing other foods while your new babies are growing inside. Also, because you select the strongest seedlings to transplant, you are likely to have higher success.

You can also buy your starts. Sometimes I love the instant gratification of going to the garden store, buying a bunch of starts, transplanting them in the big garden, and bam! Garden happens. When buying starts, don't choose the biggest, gangly ones because they're more likely to be "root bound." Their roots have grown so much they are circling themselves in the pot. It is perfectly okay to check for this while you're shopping: tip the plant and pot over, using your fingers to hold the soil surface in place, gently lift the pot off the soil ball, and look at the root system. When planting store-bought starts, keep in mind that most small plants don't like to be handled by their stems. They prefer to be moved by their entire soil root ball (after you've turned them upside down and removed the pot), or they can be picked up out of loosened soil by their leaves.

Whether you grow your own starts or buy them, the most important thing about transplanting is to be sure to water the plant right after you put it in the ground.

Seeding

There are times when seeding out in the garden does make sense. The "big seeds" like beans, corn, and potatoes are super-easy crops to direct-seed into the ground. They don't like to be transplanted anyway, so you might as well direct-seed.

A technique called "broadcast seeding" works well for the really smaller seeds such as leaf lettuces, greens, radishes, turnips, and carrots. To broadcast seed, simply mark off the area where you want the vegetable to grow, and sprinkle, or broadcast, the seeds as uniformly across the area as you can. Then lightly tamp down the soil and water the seeds. These smaller, more tender seeds need to be watered at least twice daily to keep them moist enough while they sprout.

Broadcast seeding also comes with the job of thinning. Because you are likely to have far too many plants for optimal spacing, you'll need to thin some out. This can be emotionally difficult for new gardeners, but I suggest you think of it as growing sprouts. Too many radishes or turnips in an area? Simply pull out the excess ones, thank them for growing, and pop them in your mouth for a quick snack.

seed depth guide

How deep should you plant your seeds? This varies from plant to plant, but a good general rule is to plant the seeds twice as deep as they are long. Some tiny seeds, such as lettuce, need light to germinate. They should be placed directly on top of the soil and covered with a shallow dusting of soil, but not so much that it completely blocks out the light.

Spacing

Some plants get much bigger than others, and spacing is important to keep in mind. To help with this, do yourself a favor and pick up a copy of John Jeavons's book, *How to Grow More Vegetables (and Fruits, Nuts, Berries, Grains, and Other Crops) Than You Ever Thought Possible on Less Land with Less Water Than You Can Imagine*. It will be useful to you, not only as a beginner but throughout all the years and decades of your gardening life. Gardeners owe a great debt of gratitude to Jeavons. He created a whole system for growing, but my favorite parts of the book are the detailed tables on all the common food crops, including the optimal plant spacing distance. Jeavons innovated the concept of planting in a hexagonal, or intensive, pattern to maximize the number of plants you can fit into a small space—a much more efficient method than traditional row planting. In addition, by growing at the optimal closeness, the plants crowd out weeds, keeping your weeding chores to a minimum.

The following table gives recommended plant spacings in a garden using hexagonal planting. Coincidentally, these numbers also reflect the approximate diameter of the plant.

Do bear in mind that with intensive plantings, the plants use the minerals in the soil more quickly, so you'll need to add compost and fertilizer regularly—definitely after each season, and often a handful or two or three during the growing cycle. (I have a lot more to say about fertilizer in Chapter 5.)

recommended plant spacings

Plant	Inches	Plant	Inches
Asparagus	15 to 18	Lettuce, head	10 to 12
Beans, bush	4 to 6	Lettuce, leaf	4 to 6
Beans, lima	4 to 6	Melons	18 to 24
Beans, pole	6 to 12	Mustard	6 to 9
Beets	2 to 4	Okra	12 to 18
Broccoli	12 to 18	Onions	2 to 4
Brussels sprouts	15 to 18	Peas, black-eyed	3 to 4
Cabbage	15 to 18	Peas, sugar snap or English	2 to 4
Cabbage, Chinese	10 to 12	Peppers	12 to 15
Carrots	2 to 3	Potatoes	10 to 12
Cauliflower	15 to 18	Pumpkins	24 to 36
Chard, Swiss	6 to 9	Radishes	2 to 3
Collards	12 to 15	Rutabaga	4 to 6
Cucumbers	12 to 18	Spinach	4 to 6
Eggplant	18 to 24	Squash, summer	16 to 24
Endive	15 to 18	Squash, winter	24 to 36
Garlic	3 to 4	Strawberries	8 to 12
Kale	15 to 18	Sweet corn	15 to 18
Kohlrabi	6 to 9	Tomatoes	18 to 24
Leeks	3 to 6	Turnips	4 to 6

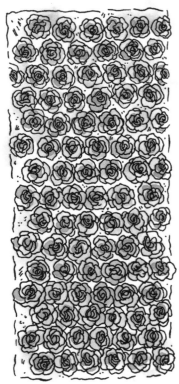

INTENSIVE HEXAGONAL
PLANT SPACING

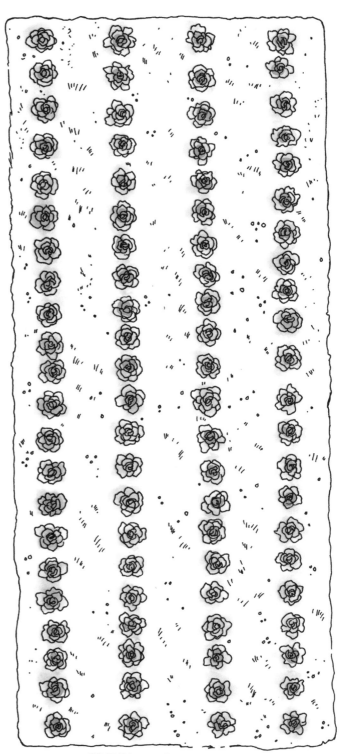

TRADITIONAL ROW SPACING

the best crops for beginners

If you are a beginner gardener, here are some crops that are easy to start with:

- **Beans**
- **Carrots**
- **Garlic**
- **Kale**
- **Lettuces**
- **Potatoes**
- **Radishes**
- **Snap peas**
- **Squash**
- **Strawberries**
- **Turnips**

Kids often love to help with strawberries and snap peas, so if you have children, try planting those crops to get your family involved. Kale and lettuces also have the advantage of being "cut and come again" crops that keep producing throughout the season.

Take It *Slooooooow*

It can be really dispiriting to watch all your hard work shrivel up and die because you've overwhelmed your garden. If this is your first time gardening, I highly recommend you start with just three or four items. Leafy greens are easy to grow and produce quickly, giving you a confidence boost. Squashes, radishes, and beans are also very easy and quick. I know you probably want to grow tomatoes, and please do go for it, but know that tomatoes are a surprisingly finicky crop. Even very experienced gardeners don't always get the tomato crop they would like, so don't worry if your tomatoes aren't as productive as you hoped. (Be sure to grow something else that's a sure winner along with your tomatoes, so you still have some crops to harvest.) Or consider a small herb garden to start with. Mint, parsley, basil, oregano, and thyme are great herbs to get you going. Mint in particular is very hardy and grows abundantly.

What to Plant When?

This is *the* gardening question: What should you plant when? Predicting the weather has always been a challenge, and it is even more so today. And of course, temperature and precipitation vary across the country and around the globe. What's even more complicated is the fact that weather patterns all over the planet are increasingly unpredictable. Still, I can give you some basic guidelines and suggestions for resources to help you no matter where you live.

All questions about the best growing seasons center around the temperature at which water freezes: 32 degrees Fahrenheit. There are two things related to freezing you need to know: what plants can still live when the temperature drops below freezing, and what the frost dates are in your region.

Cool Season vs. Warm Season Crops

A neighbor who was a newbie homesteader called me over one November to look at her dead squash plants. She was mystified as to why they had died. "We had a frost last night," I told her, "and squash dies below freezing." "But," she told me, "that package said they were *winter* squash." I gently explained to her that "winter squash" meant you grow it in the summer, like all squash, but it can be stored and eaten throughout the winter, whereas "summer squash" has to be eaten fresh. The name indicates when you can *eat* it, not when you *plant* it.

On the other hand, some plants *can* grow in the winter (but not winter squash—although you can see why she was confused!). Garden plants are roughly divided into cool season crops and warm season crops. As you can probably guess, cool season crops can withstand, and actually enjoy, colder temperatures, and warm season crops need heat to produce. There is a lot of overlap in the two categories, and what might be a cool season crop in the Southern United States may be a warm season crop in the northern part of the country.

a correlation between
civilization and plant growth?

In his book *Guns, Germs, and Steel: The Fates of Human Societies*, Jared Diamond makes a very compelling case that technology and civilization spread more quickly throughout Europe and Asia because those land masses are largely along the same east-west axis. With the same latitude comes similar temperature ranges, and food crops can be moved and adapted easily. Development of a species in one area can be transferred to another area quickly, and easier access to food meant more time could be devoted to developing new technologies. In the Americas, our continents are largely along a north-south axis, and plant species take much longer to adapt to different temperature zones, if they adapt at all, so it was much more difficult to share development of food crops among regions.

One of the reasons I created The Grow Network is so backyard researchers and experimenters all over the world can connect online to share tips and find inspiration. For example, all the people who live in the temperate regions on the planet share the same challenges regardless of whether they live in Uruguay, Eastern China, Europe, or the Eastern United States. With our rapidly changing world, we need to increase the speed and availability of sharing information on how to live resiliently, especially when it comes to home-scale agriculture, where the wisdom is often hard-won over years of experimenting and trial and error.

The following lists include plants that like it cool and those that like it hot. Bear in mind these lists are greatly affected by where you live. When I first started growing food in Colorado, I was afraid to plant lettuce because I didn't believe it would grow in the summer. I was emotionally scarred from the years of homesteading in Texas, where lettuce would burn to a crisp by June. But in Colorado, lettuce grows great all summer long, and I had delicious salads even while the sun was high in the sky. All summer, I kept pinching myself to be sure I wasn't dreaming. (I think there could be a whole branch of psychology dedicated to therapists who help you get over gardening traumas.)

Cool Season Crops That Can Handle a Frost

Asparagus	Leeks
Broccoli	Onions
Brussels sprouts	Peas
Cabbage	Radishes
Collards	Rhubarb
Fava beans	Shallots
Garlic	Spinach
Horseradish	Sunflower seeds
Kale	Turnips
Kohlrabi	

Crops That Like It Cool but Need Protection from Frost

Beets	Endive
Cauliflower	Lettuce
Celery	Mustard
Chard	Parsnips
Chinese cabbage	Potatoes
Cilantro	Swiss chard

Crops That Like It Warmer

Basil

Beans

Black-eyed peas

Cantaloupe

Corn

Cucumbers

Eggplant

Green beans

Honeydew melons

Malabar spinach

New Zealand spinach

Okra

Peppers

Pumpkins

Squash

Sweet potatoes

Tomatoes

Watermelon

Yardlong beans

These lists are a great general guideline, but there are some really unique exceptions folks have created by experimenting. (I talk about these exciting possibilities in Chapter 11.)

Frost Windows and Other Variables

Along with knowing what crops usually do well in freezing temperatures and what crops like the heat, you also need to know when the first and last frost dates are in your region. Knowing your frost window is imperative, but this is a variable that is difficult to pinpoint. Most people talk about the averages, and that is the best place to start, but be prepared for almost anything around those dates.

Predicting weather patterns and knowing when there will be a frost (or not) has always been a subject of contemplation for growers. Pairing it with observing wind patterns, clouds, the movement of birds, and the behavior of the wildlife used to be a common activity. Discussing the weather with an elder who had been making such observations all their life was a serious conversation that could give you incredible insights into the rhythms of nature. But sadly, most of those observant elders are long gone. Talking about the weather has dwindled from a source of great wisdom to more superficial conversation for most.

People often ask me my opinion on climate change and weather modification as it pertains to backyard food production. I've flown across the United States, from New York to San Francisco, on a bright, clear, moonlit night. After we crossed the eastern mountain range, I saw only circles and squares of irrigation pivots and fields of crops below me for the entire trip to the front range of Colorado. Little land was left uncultivated. Humans can have, and are having, a big impact on the planet and its weather.

The way I see it, we are living through the change of an epoch on a global scale never before experienced in history, and I see today's erratic weather as a reflection of our collective turmoil during this tremendous upheaval. Predicting the weather has never been easy, and it's probably going to be even more difficult for the foreseeable future.

You're not without resources, though. Find or create a local gardening club, and get to know people who have been growing food in your area for years. They will have insights and techniques for dealing with your specific climate. Get a sense of the historical averages of first and last freezes for your region, know what temperatures the crops you are planting can withstand, and do your best.

If you do your best, it will be good enough.

The Secrets to a Green Thumb

"I hate you," Charlie said to me. "You are like my grandmother. You can make anything grow." Charlie was a powerful woman who was normally laser focused on work and taking her impressively big company to higher levels. She had grown up in a small pueblo in Mexico, and as a child, she was ashamed when her *abuela* (grandmother) would snip a cutting from a neighbor's plant, wrap it in a wet napkin, and stuff it into her pocket. Those cuttings would grow into amazing medicinal plants, beautiful flowers, and delicious foods in chipped pots, rusty coffee cans, and other random containers. After all those years of running from her past, Charlie was realizing how deeply she had admired her grandmother and wished she could be like her.

"I can show you, Charlie. It's easier than you think," I told her.

I firmly believe anyone can have a green thumb. Even if you have killed everything you tried to grow in the past, you can still succeed. People who seem to have everything grow around them magically are not supernaturally gifted or sprinkled with stardust. A green thumb really amounts to developing some easily learned habits and understanding a few basic principles. Start working on those, and I promise, not only will things grow, magic will come.

The following sections offer some tips to get you started and keep you going.

Plan in Advance

Sketching out your garden ahead of time (perhaps in your new gardening journal!—more on that coming up) accomplishes two great things: it helps you get organized and also realistic about how many seeds or starts you are going to need (helping prevent spontaneous splurges at the local nursery), and it provides a record of what you planted that year. As time goes by, you'll want to look back to see what you planted where and how well it did.

One of my first gardening teachers was a wonderful gentleman named Butch Tindell with the Ploughshare Institute for Sustainable Culture. On the first morning of the class, he told us he was going to give us the secret to a hugely successful garden. The other students and I shifted eagerly as Butch reached into a big cardboard box and pulled out clipboards with paper. As Butch handed one to each of us, he told us that keeping records and referring to them regularly would be the fastest way to becoming a prolific producer. He was right. I still have gardening notebooks from 15 years ago, and I treasure them almost like family photo albums.

start a gardening journal

You can start your gardening journal in a notebook, on your computer, or even on your smartphone, thanks to apps that can help. Record what you planted and when you planted it, when your vegetables came in, and any other notes that might help you next season, such as first and last frost and freeze dates, any unusual weather patterns you experienced, any pest problems you encountered, or any overly bountiful harvests you didn't expect.

Keep an Eye on Your Plants

Develop the habit of looking at your plants every day. Even if you only have a moment, leave your phone in the house, go outside, deeply inhale the fresh air, feel the sunshine on your face, and move gracefully with the knowledge that you are doing the most meaningful work of your day. How do the plants look? Are they pale or rich green? Are there any blotches or holes in the leaves? Look on the undersides of the leaves—do you see any insects or eggs? Stick your finger into the soil—is it moist down past your first knuckle?

Cup your hands around some leaves or the flowers, breathe on them, and then smell the plant. Plants love the carbon dioxide in your exhaled breath and some respond by intensifying their fragrances.

I recommend hand-watering to give you more time every day to look at your plants. It only takes about 2 minutes to hand-water 50 square feet, and it gives you the opportunity to notice what is going on in your garden.

Focus on Your Soil

Soil is much, much more than something that keeps your plants upright. Great soil reduces your watering needs, combats insect problems, and produces more delicious food as your tongue recognizes real nutrition that comes from the mineral content that ultimately comes from the soil. (As I mentioned before, because soil is so important, I have a lot more to say about it in Chapter 5.)

Devote 10 Minutes a Day

A 100-square-foot garden should only take about 10 minutes of tending per day on average. Yes, there will be times, such as during the initial setup and between seasons, when you'll need to put in some hours on the weekend. But most of the time, there is just not that much to do except water, observe, and love. Expect to spend about 40 percent of your time setting up and planting, 20 percent doing maintenance, and 40 percent harvesting.

When you have a failure—and you will, I promise—see what you can learn from it, and plant again. It is very rare to get 100 percent of what you planted.

Make It a Family Activity

You can bring the kids to the garden at any time, but harvest is always a sure winner. One of my fondest memories is digging potatoes with my family. We had contests to see who could find the biggest one, the smallest one, the funniest-looking one. . . . (We found one that looked just like Uncle Frank!)

Grow What You Love

Plants are sentient beings, and they respond to love. If you love pizza, grow tomatoes, peppers, onions, and basil. Who doesn't love cold, sweet, crunchy, juicy watermelon on a hot summer day? Or the taste of humble joy in mashed potatoes and green beans? Or fresh cucumbers picked off the vine with a sweetness you'll never experience from a grocery store cuke? If you love beer, you could grow barley and hops and start brewing your own. (When you do, send me a few pints.)

Talk or sing to your plants. They are astonishingly nonjudgmental and great listeners. My friend Laura grows big, beautiful flowers that radiate life. We both believe the amazing vibrancy is because she sings to her plants every day.

Is There an App for That?

Could we develop robots or sensors to help determine optimal plant species, watering requirements, and fertilization and other needs that would be helpful to beginning growers? What about apps that could tell us when to plant, weed, or harvest?

Some weeding robots are being developed right now, believe it or not, and they look like they could work well for certain styles of gardening. But if you use the intensive raised beds I recommend, there is very little weeding that needs to be done. And "garden yoga" is great for you. When I feel my body get stiff and need to stretch, the bending and flexing I do while tugging out garden intruders or checking for plant problems is just what I need. The interactive part of tending my garden fits perfectly with my lifestyle. Automation could help with watering, but again, it only takes a short time to water, and it's a good ritual to get you outside, looking and interacting with your plants.

That said, a lot of software is being developed for garden planning, timing, and more. These programs are moving from somewhat crude to sophisticated interactive software platforms. I'm definitely watching them, but I'll confess that I love my good old paper notebook. In it, I have my garden layout and my planting guide. I have some tables for conversions, plant spacing, and other references. I have a place for notes and a log for keeping track of harvests. It's also a good place to stash some favorite recipes.

In your first years of gardening, you won't need to worry about rotating plants, but as you advance, it may become a concern. I love having the previous years' notebooks handy to quickly review what happened before. Maybe I'll change my mind later, but for now, I love the old-fashioned way of keeping track. Besides, I spend too much time looking at screens, so writing in a journal is a good thing for me. I suppose it is a personal preference.

into the future with ai?

I was privileged to interview Dr. Kai-Fu Lee, one of the world's leading experts on artificial intelligence (AI) and author of the book *AI Superpowers: China, Silicon Valley, and the New World Order*, who is sometimes called the "Bill Gates of China" for his accumulated wealth and influence. Dr. Lee also told me his family always had a garden, often tended by his brother. Especially when they first moved to the United States, he and his family longed for the tastes of vegetables they could not find in American stores, so they grew them themselves.

I asked Dr. Lee if he saw AI-powered robots or control centers helping guide the many new people who would be growing food in the coming years, and he sighed and said no, that there aren't enough data points to create something like that because each backyard and situation is different and unique.

We also discussed the tsunami of unemployment now hitting us as AI takes over more and more jobs that used to be done by humans. I proposed that if one person was designated to grow food for the whole family, it was probably better financially than having a job. The savings in groceries and medical costs could be equivalent to one well-paying salary. Dr. Lee agreed this could be part of the solution. "But," he insisted, "only if the person growing the food loves doing it."

I couldn't agree more.

Connecting with Our Past—Heirloom Varieties

Homesteaders often called springtime the "starving times" because so little food was available. The winter stores were getting low or were completely depleted, and the new crops were just being planted. In this spring food gap, homesteaders yearned to still have nice, big, fat squashes, potatoes, or other vegetables that hadn't molded.

Squashes didn't develop great storage lives on their own. Perhaps it was your great-great-grandmother who helped develop a line of squash that tasted wonderful and was a "good keeper," which meant it could be stored for many months in a root cellar or under the bed.

Over time, and with careful tending from humans, most of our common garden vegetables have sacrificed their own defenses; reduced bitter or toxic aspects; and focused their energy on larger fruits, tubers, or flowers. They would never do these things on their own, in a wild state, without human intervention. They now depend on their human gardeners to plant, protect, feed, and save their seeds so they can be propagated again.

It is a long process of growing the plants and then selecting the seeds from those plants that have the most desirable characteristics. In most of the world, you can only grow a crop once per year, so the development of a "good keeper" heirloom took many decades, if not centuries, to create.

When you hold a packet of heirloom seeds in your hands, you are holding a legacy of relationships between people and plants. As you start growing your own food, you'll find yourself tapping into that relationship, too. It's a beautiful dance to be a part of.

I love to sit in the middle of my growing corn patch. My heart rate slows, my breath deepens, and my belly calms with the primal knowledge that it will be full that coming winter. Corn absolutely cannot grow without humans, and humans need the corn to eat to stay alive and be healthy. The corn knows this, and when you sit in your own corn patch and be still, you will feel it, too.

Heirlooms Just Taste Better

You can't put a price on the food you grow yourself, and you can't buy anything that tastes better. I found this out firsthand after tasting just how much better my own homegrown food was—even better than the best local organic farmer.

One year, I was living in the Rocky Mountains of Colorado. I wasn't familiar with gardening in such a cold climate, so I asked Lynn Gillespie of The Living Farm to be my gardening coach. Not only is Lynn a gardening instructor, but she also runs a small community supported agriculture (CSA) to feed her local community. Lynn grows the produce for her CSA in the same raised bed gardening system she teaches to backyard gardeners. After more than 30 years of growing, Lynn has really dialed in a simple system for how to grow food.

We set up two raised beds in my yard and filled them with Lynn's secret soil recipe.

I used the exact same everything in my yard that Lynn uses in her growing system. I had the same raised beds, her soil, her plants, her seeds, her timing, and her fertilizers. Lynn only lives a few miles from me, so even the climate was the same. Everything I had was identical to what Lynn uses in her CSA.

Because I have so many friends, family, coworkers, and other interesting people in my life, I generally need a lot more food than you might think. So in addition to growing food in my own raised beds, I signed up for Lynn's CSA. What can I say? I want to be sure those close to me eat well, and I love throwing big parties where I can feed them.

Lynn is an extremely talented organic farmer, and her vegetables are amazing. But I can tell you that the vegetables I grew myself—after interacting with them every day, talking to them, watering them, and caring for them—just tasted better.

The food you grow yourself is priceless.

biological intelligence

I've been absolutely delighted to see that the connection growing things have with each other is no longer considered as "out there" as it once was, but is actually becoming the focus of serious scientific research. Monica Gagliano at the University of Western Australia is a researcher in the new field of biological intelligence. Gagliano developed a series of experiments in which she trained pea plants to respond to stimuli very much as Pavlov did with his dogs. Not only did the plants learn, but they also remembered.

The book *The Hidden Life of Trees: What They Feel, How They Communicate—Discoveries from a Secret World* by Peter Wohlleben is all about the latest research into tree intelligence. I always wondered why deer and other herbivores continually move as they eat. Why don't the deer just stay in one place and eat there longer? It turns out from the scientific research Wohlleben brings forward that a tree knows when it's being eaten, and it quickly changes the tastes of its leaves to be unpalatable to the deer. The even more amazing aspect of his research is that the tree also communicates to its nearby "friends and family" about the intruder, and they all change the taste of their leaves. The deer seem to know the distance and move to the next tree that is out of range of the local communication network. And that is why deer and other browsers continually move. There is so much more going on in a forest than any of us ever imagined!

Homegrown Food on Every Table

One of the biggest successes a new group of gardeners ever had was during World War II, when 20 million novice American gardeners turned their lawns into gardens, and in the first year, grew 40 percent of the produce consumed in the United States.

Most people think the Victory Garden movement was a WWII initiative, but Loretta Craig, a Kansas farmer and Victory Garden enthusiast, points out that it actually began prior to WWI in response to food shortages. There were food riots in

America in the early 1900s, and the "grow your own food" movement was created by a grassroots group of citizens to help prevent further civil unrest.

Could we do that today? Absolutely. And the great news is, most of the infrastructure is already in place.

According to a study from NASA scientists in collaboration with researchers in the Mountain West, an estimated total of 40 million acres of lawns in America are already set up with irrigation. It is a bizarre factoid that grass is the United States' largest irrigated crop. In fact, it is three times more prevalent than any other irrigated crop in the country. Based on my estimates, we could feed all 330 million Americans if individuals and families worked these 40 million acres of irrigated lawns.

And for you urbanites, did you know that Manhattan has 14,000 acres of rooftop space with enough sunlight and structural integrity to hold gardens? Laurie Schoeman, director of New York Sun Works, a nonprofit group that promotes growing food on rooftops, says that if all those roofs had greenhouses, the resulting produce could feed up to 20 million people in the New York area.

Although there is tremendous nutrition in your garden, the *process* of growing food may be healthier than the products—the gentle movements, the fresh air, the sunshine, the family connections, and the stress reduction. These are the keys to health and longevity. This is real wealth.

I really appreciate my local farmers, but once you get good at growing your own produce, no amount of money can buy anything that is as tasty or nutritious as food you have grown yourself in rich soil and tended with love.

some fun foods to grow

Sure, part of having a garden is producing high-quality, great-tasting, super-nutritious foods . . . and part of it is just for fun! Check out some of these foods you'll want to grow just for the heck of it.

Cherry tomatoes. These are so sweet and hugely prolific. Just like candy, really.

Beets. You can get kids to eat a lot of red beets if you tell them their poop will come out red. They'll do it just to see it.

Sunflowers. The huge flower heads move each day to track the sun, starting in the east in the morning, moving to the west by the end of the day, and then nodding down at night. It's amazing to watch. Roasted, salted sunflower seeds are a yummy treat, too.

Asparagus. Boys especially will eat a lot of this if you tell them their pee will smell funny. When serving asparagus, slather it with butter and garlic.

Popping corn. Corn is wind pollinated and needs some room to grow (it will take up all of your 100 square feet), but it is such a fun treat and makes great gifts.

Mint. Most members of the mint family are very hardy once they get established. In fact, you may have a tough time getting rid of it. Mints smell wonderful and make delightful tea. You can even candy the leaves as a special treat for kids or visitors.

Cubical watermelons. Okay, this is a little crazy, but I have this strange desire to grow a cubical watermelon. Doesn't that just sound like fun?

chapter summary

- Your taste buds will discover new universes when you start growing your own food.

- A 50-square-foot raised bed is the perfect size for a beginner.

- Transforming a black thumb to green is easy.

- Food you have grown yourself, in rich soil and tended with love, is priceless.

additional resources

For more information on backyard gardening, check out these websites:

- www.GrowHalf.com. A short, inspiring video that shows you a simple, three-part system for how to grow half of your own food in your backyard. It includes exactly what you can produce, how much time it takes, how many calories are created, and what it is like to operate on a day-to-day basis.

- www.HighPerformanceGardening.com. Watch over our shoulders as Lynn Gillespie and I take you through an entire season of growing food—starting with an untouched lawn, constructing the beds, working the soils, planting, tending, dealing with pests and predators, and harvesting. We also do a lot of joking around. Well, I do a lot of joking around, and Lynn worries about me. But it's fun to binge-watch the entire season, and you'll see how two experienced gardeners grow food.

- www.GardenerQuiz.com. What personalities make the best gardeners, and what type are you? Find out your gardening personality type with this fun quiz.

- www.Seeds2Sauce.com. Everything you wanted to know about tomatoes but were afraid to ask . . . This bundle of videos is curated from my years of hosting online summits with tomato-growing experts.

chapter 3

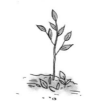

the eggs:
easily grow 365 breakfasts and
dozens of deviled eggs

He watched the sun dropping toward the horizon and knew he would be dead soon. After dark, all manner of predators come out: raccoons, bobcats, foxes, and coyotes. Everyone likes to eat chickens. He struggled again, but it was useless; his wings and legs were completely bound up in the flexible fencing.

That is when I came upon him. On my way to handle afternoon chores, I saw that Buddy, my big, beautiful, black rooster, had accidentally gotten himself stuck in some portable fencing. Normally the flock is quite self-reliant, and the chickens know about the fence, but no system is 100 percent foolproof, and Buddy was in trouble. I slowed down as I walked toward Buddy and very gently disentangled him. When I released him, he shook for a moment, resettling all his feathers. He must have been there for a while because the next thing he did was run to get some water. Then he went straight to the flock, won a fight with the junior rooster, and reestablished his place as leader of the flock.

I didn't think much of it after that, except to be glad that I had walked by and saved a really good rooster.

Then the next day, something happened I will never forget. I was working in the orchard in an open area, weeding a young sapling. It was about midday and Texas hot. At that time of day, the chickens (who are probably smarter than I am) lounge under a shade tree, take dust baths, and rest well away from the beating sun. So I was surprised when Buddy came walking right up to where I was sitting on the ground, out in the open sun, working. He stood in front of me just out of arm's length, and for a long moment, he stared directly at me. (Because chickens' eyes are on the sides of their heads, his stare was in a side-eyed chicken sort of way.) When he was sure he had my attention, he started to slowly walk in a perfect circle all around me. After he completed his circle, he stopped in front of me again, scratched at the ground a few times with his head lowered but his eye on me, stood up erect again, and walked away.

No chicken has ever done anything like that before, or since, and I knew it was his way of saying thank you. Even as I write this, so many years later, the memory still brings tears to my eyes.

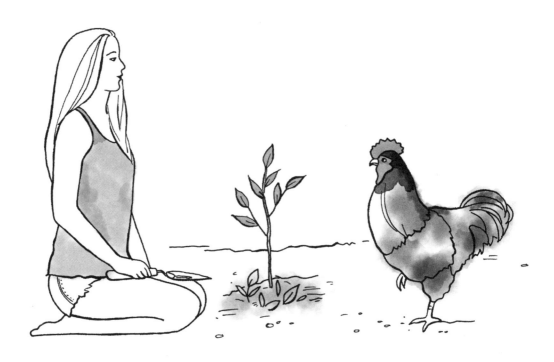

Almost everyone who keeps chickens experiences delightful relationships with their birds—many even half-jokingly refer to their chickens as "pets with benefits."

The benefits are incredible. Chickens create an abundant source of protein that does not require much effort from you after you get them started. And if you care about where your food comes from, raising your own hens can give you strong peace of mind. Trying to decipher the labels used on commercially produced eggs—cage-free, free-range, vegetarian, organic, pasteurized, fertilized—can be baffling. But with your own hens, you'll know exactly what they've eaten and how they've been cared for—a fact that will make you feel good about the eggs you feed your family.

At the same time, as I did with Buddy and many other chickens in my flock over the years, you are likely to discover a real sense of purpose in caring for your animals and providing them with a healthy, productive, and environmentally sustainable way of life.

therapy chickens

A friend of mine has a daughter who was adopted out of foster care. She was born with methamphetamine in her system, and when she was very young, she suffered from terrible fits of anger. It just so happened that the family owned some chickens. One friendly little golden hen named Honey became the little girl's therapy chicken. Anytime she got upset, she would go outside to hold her little hen, and she would calm right down.

This family isn't alone. Many people are discovering how raising chickens can provide a release from the stresses of modern life. The next time you feel anxious or depressed, try cuddling a chicken.

Mount *Egg-erest*: The Ultimate Superfood

A good laying hen in her prime will lay about 250 eggs a year. If you have a small flock of six hens, that is about 1,500 eggs! Think three-egg omelets every day of the year for breakfast, plus numerous platters of deviled eggs and dozens of eggs left over to share with friends and family. Forget the bottle of wine or the cellophane-wrapped cookies—when you bring a dozen of your own fresh backyard eggs as a hostess gift, see how high your friend's eyebrows raise and how big she smiles.

Not only are chickens incredible food producers, but the eggs they create are power-packed with nutrition. What part of the fresh egg, if fertilized, would have become a chicken? If you are like most folks, you'd say "the yolk," but actually, the chicken is only a tiny, microscopic cell containing the union of DNA from the hen and the cock. The yolk is basically a big packet of food for the growing embryo.

Let's think about that for a moment. Within the yolk, and the clear albumin we often call the "white," is all the nutrition needed for a fertilized cell so tiny we can't see it with our naked eyes. That cell eventually becomes a chick, with a fully developed body and organs and enough nutritional reserves to keep it going for 3 days after it hatches. All the micro- and macronutrients, all the minerals, all the vitamins—everything needed for that miracle chicken to grow is contained primarily in the yolk. That is my definition of a superfood!

So then imagine the nutritional boost and improvement in your own health you get from eating fresh, beautiful, nutritious eggs from hens who are living a good life in your backyard. Cooked or raw, eggs are a good source of inexpensive, high-quality nutrition. They are especially good as a complete protein source. Eggs contain all eight essential amino acids, including the ones that we cannot synthesize in our bodies and must obtain from our diet.

Eggs have been in the human diet for forever, and although there's still some debate about eggs and cholesterol, I have been eating at least three eggs a day for many, many years, and my blood numbers are always fine. In fact, my life insurance company rates my health as "preferred premium," which means it's betting I will live for a long, long time.

Your Cock-a-Doodle-Don't Need a Rooster

Most people think of a crowing rooster at dawn when they imagine chickens on a farm. But I want to point out that you don't need a rooster to raise laying hens, and for city dwellers, I strongly recommend you do not have a rooster. They really are loud and can drive you, and your neighbors, crazy!

I had a good laugh once when I was visiting New York City and heard a rooster crowing. The sound ricocheted among the tightly packed buildings, so it was impossible to know exactly where it was coming from. I don't think even Google could ever find that guy! There is no telling how many New Yorkers that rooster annoyed every morning. You really do not want to be a source of annoyance in your community. Your hens will be able to lay eggs just fine without the services of the boys.

Plus, roosters can be really hard to have around. Roosters, or "cocks," generally *are* cocky. (Many idioms like this are derived from our agrarian ancestry.) Plus, some are downright mean and will harass young children. For farm kids, finally winning over the rooster is a rite of passage. My kids did learn to face their fear of our big, mean roosters, and later I found much more amenable cocks. But beware that not all birds are as gentlemanly as Buddy!

The Basic Recipe for a Backyard Flock of Laying Chickens

Ingredients
6 laying hens
1 rooster (optional)
Predator-safe coop and run
Fencing for yard access
Chicken feed and feeding system
Watering system

Choosing Your Laying Hens

There are many different breeds of chickens! The variety is both wonderful and overwhelming. Here are some basic principles that will help you be successful in picking a breed that is compatible for where you live.

First, let's take a step back. There is a rough division of birds based on their primary purpose: they are either "egg-layers" or "meat birds." When you are beginning to grow and raise your own food, it is best to focus on using hens for eggs. Eggs are a nutritious, plentiful, and quick food source, and you can keep the chickens in a small space. Meat chickens require more time and space and are not as productive: one meat chicken might cover a single-family dinner, but one mature laying hen will provide many, many meals' worth of eggs. So I will focus just on egg-layers in this chapter.

Picking your breed is fun! With so many breeds to choose from, you are likely to have several favorites. When people ask me my favorite breed, I feel like they are asking me to choose between my children. (Okay, if I'm honest, I'll confess there are some days when I know exactly which one of my kids I like better . . . but let's not go there.)

Chickens are quite versatile and can adapt to most conditions, but a great starting point for selecting a breed is to consider what birds are more adapted to your climate. Egg-laying does slow down in winter as a chicken's hormonal systems respond to the decreasing daylight hours. But if a chicken is having trouble keeping itself warm, egg production will completely stop. Conversely, if a hen is overheated and miserable, egg production also drops.

The basic anatomy of a bird makes it more suitable for certain climates. The chickens' combs and wattles (those fleshy parts on the top of their head and under their chins) are especially useful for dissipating heat. Large wattles and combs also have a greater tendency of getting frostbitten. So in warmer climates, you want birds with big wattles and combs, and in colder climates, you want birds with smaller ones. Note that anatomy will not compensate for poor coop design—you still need to provide proper shelter for them—but it does give your birds an edge.

The general weight of the bird also impacts its happiness in different climates. Very slight birds with less body mass do better in warmer climates, while heavier, more stout ladies are more comfortable walking through snow.

I've found that almost all chickens are good foragers, but some have a reputation for being better at it. A really good forager probably isn't the best choice for your first backyard flock, though. Their bodies tend to be very slight and angular, and they are good flyers, which means they are difficult to keep in a coop or fenced in. Great foragers are often more skittish, too, because they need to be much more alert and attuned to potential predators.

Now for temperament. All chicken breeds can be tamed with enough time and patience, but some have a predisposition for becoming friends with humans. Of course, treats such as mealworms, table scraps, or sunflower seeds really accelerate the process!

The Best Breeds for Beginners

Here is a selection of the basic, "you can't go wrong" breeds:

- **Easter Eggers.** According to the American Poultry Association, Easter Eggers aren't an official breed, but they are common and popular in many backyard flocks. Their name comes from their tendency to produce blue- and green-tinted eggs. These petite little birds have small beaks and adorable cheek feathers. They are adaptable to most climates but don't do well at the extremes of heat or cold. Easter Eggers are an especially good choice if you are going to have little kids tending the flock. Laying roughly 250 eggs per year each, they are an excellent all-around chicken and a great starter flock.

- **Orpingtons.** These ladies have the sweetest dispositions. I am most familiar with the buff Orpingtons, but they also come in lavender, blue, black, and white. With smaller wattles and stouter bodies, they are cold-hardy birds, but they've done well for me in Texas, too. They lay a respectable 200 or so white-shelled eggs each per year.

- **Barred Rocks.** I have really enjoyed the many Barred Rocks I've had in my flocks over the years. They are super easy to tame, very friendly, and inquisitive. I sometimes think they are secret comedians—my Barred Rocks have made me laugh so many times with their curious antics. They are a good all-around chicken with regard to climate. I have found Barred Rocks to be good foragers without the skittish temperament of some other chickens. They are also good layers, producing approximately 250 light brown eggs each per year.

Brahmas. These birds are famous for being gentle giants. They are very large chickens, and almost every inch of them is feathered. Although their production of about 150 large, light brown eggs each per year is not as high as other breeds, their affectionate nature and ability to lay well into colder temperatures make them a favorite with northern chicken keepers. Some folks suggest keeping a few in the flock to ensure longer availability of eggs in the winter.

Leghorns. Leghorns are the champions of egg production. There is a legend that a white Leghorn hen produced 364 eggs one year; 280 to 300 eggs per year is more reasonable. They also have a reputation for being excellent foragers and are a bit more wary, so it may take some extra time and handfuls of treats to tame them. They do well in hot climates, too. A dear elder friend of mine who grew up in West Texas during the Great Depression and through WWII told me he never saw anyone keeping all the fancy chickens. Back then, the only birds people kept in their yards were brown Leghorns.

Australorp. The Australorp is a chicken created in Australia primarily from the stock of Orpingtons and Leghorns. They have the very sweet nature of the Orpington and the egg-laying capability of the Leghorns. Buddy the rooster was a black Australorp. Black is the classic color, but there are also blue and white variations. They have good heat tolerance, thanks to their big wattles and combs, and the hens produce about 250 brown eggs each per year.

I'd like to make a quick note here that the color of the eggshell does not indicate anything about the nutritional content of the egg. Brown, blue, or speckled shells are not necessarily nutritionally different than white. What the hen ate determines the nutrient density of the egg. But it sure is delightful to see the surprise on a friend's face when he or she opens your gift of a carton full of different-colored eggs.

Why You Need Six Hens

Chickens are flocking creatures, and like other herd animals, they feel safer in a group. They experience stress just like humans do, and so you want to help them be as comfortable as possible. When you get your flock of chickens, you'll notice that when they go out foraging, almost always one of the birds has its head up to watch out for predators or other trouble. The rest of the flock will have their heads down because that is where the bugs and seeds are. From what I've noticed, they rotate this duty fairly evenly if it's a group of hens. If there is a rooster, he will be watching most of the time, which gives the hens extra time to eat. That is one reason to have a rooster if you live far enough away from other people. But hens will just as easily trade guard duty.

When you have a flock size of six hens, each hen gets a reasonable amount of time to safely scratch and peck, which creates an overall sense of security. But the fewer birds you have—say you get down to two—the longer the time each hen has to be on guard duty. Having only one hen is very cruel. Having six hens also gives you some buffer for loss. There will be times when you lose a hen or two to predators, injury, or just life.

I predict that once you get into having a flock, your love for keeping birds will grow and you'll end up with far more than six!

Counting Your Chickens after They Hatch

Although it sounds wonderful, and it definitely is fun, I don't recommend raising your birds from chicks for your first flock. Raising chicks to maturity requires a different set of skills, additional equipment, and a lot more time. (Although after you gain some experience with your flock and know the ropes, raising chicks to sell as laying hens can be a good side business.) Instead, I recommend buying some hens who are already laying so you can start collecting eggs right away. Hens start laying at about 5 months of age, they hit their prime in their second year, and they continue laying with about a 10 percent drop-off for many years onward.

Where is the best place to get your hens? Craigslist, feed stores, and local meetup groups are great places. Also, ask around at local farmers markets. I like buying directly from a local breeder so I get to see her operation and what she feeds her chickens, and I can ask for advice on the specifics of what to look out for in our region. Plus, I make a new chicken-loving friend I can call on if trouble arises.

Habitats for Hens

After you have figured out what kind of chickens you want—but before you buy the chickens—you'll need to set up housing for them. There are many different ways to keep chickens. To make it easy, start out with a fixed coop, run, and controlled access to the yard. The coop and run require little space, probably much less than you imagine. A general guideline is to have, per bird, 4 square feet of coop space, a bit of room for nest boxes, and a minimum of 10 square feet of run space. So a flock of 6 hens needs 24 square feet of coop space (6×4-foot area) and 60 square feet of run space (10×6-foot area). You will want an additional 24 square feet for nest boxes, feed storage, and other bits. When you add this all up, your flock could fit in an area about the size of a parking spot.

The absolute best place to locate your coop and run is under a deciduous tree. That way, it is naturally shaded in the summer and open to the sun in the winter. The tree will love the companionship and the fertilization the flock adds to its roots. If you don't have a deciduous tree, plant one!

There are a zillion designs for chicken coops (see the link at the end of this chapter), but here are the essential design elements you want, no matter how fancy or simple you go:

Access for Maintaining

- You should be able to access both the coop and the run (two doors).

- You need easy access to collect droppings for cleaning and maintenance. Chickens poop a lot at night. This is kind of awesome, though, because it makes it easy to get the ingredients for your compost pile. *Note: Chicken manure is too "hot" to put directly on plants and needs to be composted first. Fresh or recent chicken manure has too much nitrogen and will literally burn plants if you use it.*

Nest Boxes

- You'll need two nest boxes, each one about 12 inches square. Milk crates make excellent nest boxes.

- You want to have easy access to the nest boxes from the outside.

Roosting Bar

- Have a space that's 10 inches per bird for most hens and 12 inches per bird if you have bigger breeds. So approximately 5 to 6 feet of roosting space.

- Roosts should be higher than the nests.

Ramp

- You need a ramp for the chickens to get in and out of the coop and into the run.

Ventilation

- There should be ventilation up high in the coop that includes adjustable openings to adapt for seasonal changes. You need at least two vents with 1 square foot of opening in each.

Fencing and Protection

- Use fencing around the run, and bury it at least 1 foot deep to prevent tunneling predators. Fencing for the run should be ½-inch hardware cloth or similar. You might get away with chicken wire, but I've seen chicken wire ripped apart by some seriously hungry predators.

- Use fencing on the top of the run.

- Add raccoon-proof latches. Do not underestimate the intelligence of raccoons. They are smart, athletic, and strong, and they have all night, every night, to work on the problem of how to get to your chickens.

- Add an automatic, solar-powered door to close the chickens in at night.

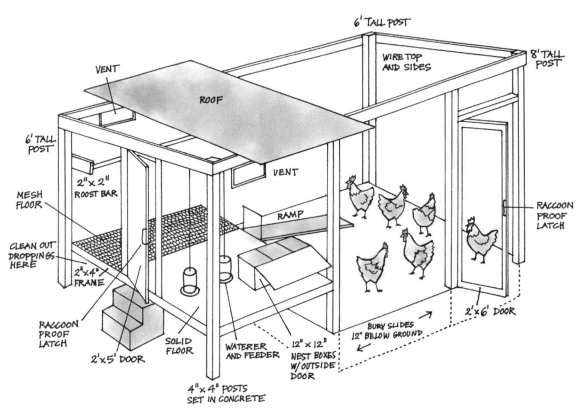

COOP AND RUN FOR 6 HENS

The chickens' run should be a fixed area that is fenced well. It is sometimes called a "sacrifice pen" because within a few days, the chickens will eat everything in the area and the ground will be bare. But it's a great safe place for your chickens to get outside and enjoy the sun, and it is an easy place for you to dump food scraps for them.

Speaking of raccoons, most people think the rural countryside is the most dangerous place to keep chickens because they think all the predators live out there, but that's not exactly true. In the burbs, wildlife is surprisingly more abundant because there are so many more food sources in a more concentrated space. Think of all the landscaped and irrigated fruit and nut trees, bird feeders, garbage pails, pet food bowls, water features with fish, and lap cats and dogs that accidentally got outside for the night. All that might be in the country, too, but it's more spread out.

Chickens on the Loose

You will want to let your chickens out of the coop and run on a regular basis. This is healthy for the chickens, it cuts down on your feed costs, and you'll never have a tick problem in your yard. To a chicken, ticks are tasty little appetizers.

But before you let your chickens loose in your yard, let's talk.

In Texas, you see a lot of cattle pens filled with a beautiful, hardy, yellow flower called the cowpen daisy. That will be the only plant in the pen. No native grasses, no amaranth, no dandelions—nothing. Just dirt and the cowpen daisy. A general principle when you keep any livestock is that they eat their favorite things first. Then their second favorite. And so on. Then it gets to the point where the only thing left is what's inedible to the animals.

I know it won't surprise you that cows really hate the taste of cowpen daisies.

To work around this, farmers rotate what areas the livestock have access to so the land can regenerate between animal visits. This is true for any size livestock, from buffalos to pigeons, and yes, chickens.

Holistic Range Management is an agricultural approach that focuses on effectively rotating animals on land to vastly increase production, fertility, and biodiversity. Properly managed grazing animals are the quickest and most effective way to restore pasture and savannahs. But how do you implement this in your yard with your chickens? Well, if your yard is big enough and your chicken flock is small, your birds may never be able to eat down all their favorites, in which case you can simply let them out and they will be fine. My rough guess is you will need ½ to 1 acre for a flock of six hens to maintain a healthy pasture. But keep in mind that variables such as climate, rainfall, growth rates, and your plantings all impact this equation.

Even if you do have a big yard, you probably won't want to give them full access anyway because chickens love to tear up the mulch around your landscaping, ravage your compost piles, and poop in places you don't want them to poop.

The best solution is to set up some portable fencing that you move around from time to time to give them access to different parts of the yard in a controlled fashion. I am a huge fan of the fencing products from Premier1Supplies. The company has portable fencing that is super easy to put up, move around, and take down, and it can be electrified with a solar charger, which both deters predators and keeps the chickens in. I once talked with a farmer who was raising large flocks of chickens in an area of Texas known as Coyote Creek. Seems like a terrible place to try to keep chickens if you ask me. I couldn't understand why all the coyotes didn't jump his fencing. But his pastured flock was always surrounded by movable electrified poultry netting, and that did the trick. The farmer told me he regularly saw coyotes sitting outside the fence drooling, but they never tried to come over it.

What about your garden? You will want to fence your garden for many reasons other than your chickens. Most of the time, you won't want your chickens in your garden, but you can let them in between seasons so they can pick at what's left, eat insects, and do a light tilling. There are only a few special occasions when I have let the chickens into my garden during the growing season. Once was when I had an infestation of some kind of beetle all over my sweet potato plants. They were the coolest-looking beetles—they were so shiny their backs reflected light like chrome. (I wondered if they might be from outer space!) But I really wanted to eat sweet potatoes, and something had to be done and quick. I let the chickens into the garden for a short while and encouraged them toward the beetles. I stayed with them for the 15 minutes or so it took the hens to eat most of the bugs and then I escorted the chickens out before they headed toward my kale. (Side note: because insect presence usually means the plants have some weakness, after escorting the chickens out, I gave the sweet potatoes some nourishing seaweed and compost tea solution to boost their overall health.)

Jere Gettle, founder of Baker Creek Heirloom Seeds, has a fenced chicken run that surrounds his garden. The idea is that the chickens patrol the perimeter and eat insects that are crossing through but don't have access to the plants. He told me he thought it helped. That's a difficult thing to determine quantitatively, but it certainly gave the chickens extra area to roam. I have seen lots of people who do an inverse sort of arrangement. They let the chickens roam about the entire yard but have several smaller island areas fenced off with limited access. You may need to go through some trial and error before you know what works best for you and your chickens.

What Does an Egg Factory Eat?

Can your chickens survive completely on what they find in your yard and perhaps some scraps you toss them? Modern chickens are all descendants of jungle fowl originating in Southeast Asia. In their natural state, they are primarily insectivores (insects contain a lot of protein and fat) who also eat greens. The closer your backyard comes to looking like Southeast Asia, the less you will need to feed your chickens. Actually, given their semitropical origins, it is amazing that chickens have adapted so well to colder climates. But the farther north you live, the more you will need to provide some of their diet.

A rough guideline is that during the growing seasons in your region, when greens and insects are abundant, your yard can provide about 30 percent of your chickens' food. There are many creative ways to get free feed for your chickens and to stretch the chicken feed you do buy. But as a beginner, you have got a lot to learn, and I strongly recommend you keep it simple and start out buying feed.

Feed

You can buy chicken feed at your local co-op or farm supply store. Look for layer feed that has at least 16 percent protein. It also should have some crushed oyster shell to supply your flock with the calcium they need for egg production. A 50-pound bag of feed should last your girls approximately 1 month.

Should you spend the extra money on all-organic feed? There is a bit of debate on this topic. Of course, an organic label provides some assurance that the feed is clean, and it also supports organic farming. But many people simply buy non–genetically modified organism (GMO) feed instead. There are two big reasons why non-GMO feed is probably going to be just fine (and a bit less expensive). First, fresh greens are known to be blood-cleansers, and if your birds are getting fresh forage every day, that can offset any potential problems in non-GMO commercial grains. Secondly, many farmers who grow non-GMO grains use practices that go beyond organic, but they don't bother with the certification. The certification process is expensive, time-consuming, and offers little reward for small farmers. Joel Salatin, known as "America's Farmer," is a prolific writer and champion for local regenerative agriculture. Salatin lists certifications as one of the top 10 expensive distractions new farmers should avoid. So many small farmers are growing clean, healthy crops but just don't bother getting certified. So try the non-GMO, but definitely avoid GMO feeds if at all possible.

Feeders

Feeders are inexpensive to buy and last many years. You can even make your own free-flow feeder for next to nothing. A free-flow feeder saves you time by automating the feeding process so all you have to do is refill the food when it gets low. Try to keep the access to the feed a bit high, because chickens are notoriously messy and wasteful if the feed is close to the ground.

Watering

You are going to need at least two watering setups. I always recommend two because having redundancy in all systems is very important. You just never know when something will break, and you don't want to stress your hens with thirst. There are lots of commercial options for waterers, or it can be a fun and easy DIY weekend project to make a couple of gravity-fed waterers out of 5-gallon buckets and float valves. Building waterers with your kids will teach them a ton of great practical science lessons.

Collecting Eggs

With your watering and feeding systems in place and a solar coop door, your chicken chores all but disappear. Most days, all you need to do is check their feed and water and collect the eggs.

Most people collect the eggs daily, but it is completely fine to skip a day or two. Don't take all the eggs from the nest, though; leave an egg or two behind. Seeing some eggs in the nest box reassures the hens the nest is active and a good place to lay. When you collect eggs is not necessarily important except that it is rude to take eggs out from under the hen while she is actively laying.

Contrary to popular belief, eggs do not need to be refrigerated. They store just fine for up to several weeks if kept cool and dark. I've found that older eggs are the best to use for hard-boiling because they are easier to peel than fresh eggs.

Historically, collecting eggs and taking care of the chickens was work small children did to help with the family food production. Starting kids early doing meaningful work and explaining the important contribution they are making to the whole family sets them up for living a life of meaning and purpose. Start them as young as possible—by the time they are teenagers, it is too late!

the poultry police

Are chickens legal in your area? If they aren't, then change the system. You have the power! I've seen it happen.

About two decades ago, keeping chickens in your backyard in Austin, Texas, was considered weird. But permaculture teacher and activist Selwyn Polit loved his birds, petitioned city hall, and was instrumental in getting city ordinances changed to allow backyard chickens. As more hens won the hearts of the city's residents, having backyard chickens started to become very popular. A yearly "funky chicken coop" tour even started so proud homeowners could show off their fancy coops and friendly flocks.

The City of Austin started to crunch some numbers. Encouraging residents to feed their food scraps to a backyard flock of chickens meant fewer truckloads of waste going to landfills. An initial study showed that if each Austinite kept a backyard flock, tons of waste could be turned into compost, and dollars would be saved. It made so much sense, it was a no-brainer decision even for a big-city bureaucracy. The City of Austin now offers residents free training for keeping backyard chickens and even a cash rebate incentive!

In New York City, the Department of Parks and Recreation now runs regular workshops on raising chickens, including tips on winterizing your coops and keeping your chickens safe from city predators like rats and dogs. So if your city is currently behind the times, don't worry. There are many examples for you to cite when approaching your local government.

Backyard chickens are so beneficial that private organizations are working to get more home flocks established. Patricia Foreman, author of the excellent book *City Chicks: Keeping Micro-Flocks of Chickens*, created the nonprofit Gossamer Foundation, which offers "Chicken Stimulus Packages" that help get folks started and become knowledgeable about family flocks. The Gossamer Foundation has given away thousands of chicks with instructions and feed, and it also maintains a hotline for first-time flock owners. Whenever I've finished a meal or meeting with Patricia, I love how instead of saying goodbye, she says "May the flock be with you."

After you get everything set up, raising chickens is almost effortless. It requires minimal time and energy and pays you back many times over with increased health and food security.

chapter summary

- Raising your own chickens gives you friendships, food security, and gifts that will raise eyebrows and generate big smiles.

- Many wonderful chicken breeds make great friendships with humans. A bird's anatomy can help you find a breed that fits your climate.

- Chickens need food and water, a coop to roost in, a run, and controlled access to a larger yard. A coop and run for six hens only require an area the size of a parking spot.

- Watering systems, feeders, and an automatic coop door cut down your workload to almost nothing.

- Eggs are a superfood.

additional resources

For more information on raising chickens, check out these websites:

- www.BackyardCoopPlans.com. Free step-by-step plans for building the perfect backyard chicken coop and run for a flock of six laying hens. Includes the parts list, 3D drawings, and modifications for different climates.

- www.FreeChickenFeed.com. A free webinar with tons of ways to get free chicken feed and lots of info on what you can and cannot feed chickens.

- www.AutomaticLivestockWaterer.com. Free step-by-step plans and a parts list for building an automatic, gravity-fed livestock waterer to automate the water needs of your flock. It doesn't need electricity!

- www.FunnyRoosterAd.com. A really funny ad for a free rooster. Please don't read this if you are easily offended.

chapter 4

the meat:
produce half the protein
for a family of four in
less than 10 minutes a day

Y ou have arrived at the chapter that will probably be the most controversial in this book. I am going to explain the value of raising, processing, and eating your own backyard meat. I do not come from a family who hunts, and I had never even thought of butchering an animal until I started homesteading. So I deeply understand all the issues that may be coming up for you.

In fact, I was a vegetarian when I started the journey to grow my own food, and I had been experimenting with being a raw vegan for a time before that. Truth be told, as an American woman, I've probably tried more diets than Oprah. We have so many choices available to us, and there is so much contradicting science and different opinions about what we should eat or not eat, it's overwhelming.

Growing my own food helped me cut through my lifelong confusion. It connected me to the past and to the way indigenous peoples who lived before us ate. I realized that, like these ancestors, I should aim to eat mostly what I can produce.

We should back up and ask the question: Just because indigenous peoples ate a particular diet, were they healthy? The simple answer to that is yes because if they weren't healthy, they would have died. The further back in history you go, the more people depended on their bodies to live. Finding or producing food, making whatever was needed, and transportation were all essential manual activities that required good hand-eye coordination, conditioning, a quick mind, and a healthy and robust body. The average member of an ancient tribe would be considered a super athlete compared to humans today.

I once visited the Tarahumara Indians of Mexico's Copper Canyon. The Tarahumara are the world's fastest long-distance runners, and they were made famous in the book *Born to Run: The Hidden Tribe, the Ultra-Runners, and the Greatest Race the World Has Never Seen* by Christopher McDougall. I met an older man named Juan Lerio, who was 71 years old. Like the other Tarahumara, Juan had a small, compact body clearly hardened by a life spent mostly outdoors.

I asked Juan about the last time he had raced. He told me had finished a 72-kilometer race the previous week. The Tarahumara like to start running at night, when it is cooler, and it took him until noon the following day to finish. I was so amazed that Juan could run so far and be in such great shape for his age. But this is common among his people. Later I would meet an 80-year-old man of equal abilities, and I was stunned at one runner named Daniel Perez, who looked so youthful at the age of 60.

Many people believe the Tarahumara are vegetarians. The staples of their diet are indeed corn, beans, and squash. So I asked Juan and the assembled group, "Do you like to eat meat?"

"Oh yes," Juan answered, with an added tone of appreciation I hadn't heard before. "What kinds of meat?" I asked. You'll get a sense of his lifestyle by the order he answered: "Squirrel, chicken, lizard, snake. . . ." Then Juan said another creature, and there was a general discussion of how to translate that into English, but no one knew. I think the closest translation is "something like a packrat."

Thinking of the cows and goat I had seen, I asked about Juan about them. "Oh yes," he and everyone agreed, they were good to eat, but rarely do they eat their herd animals. They are too valuable. The herds are needed for fertilization to grow the crops and as a form of cash. They trade goat meat with Mexicans for needed items such as tools and cloth.

So although meat is not the backbone of the Tarahumara diet, it is definitely a part of what they eat. In my research, I have found that many indigenous cultures and homesteaders living off the grid rely on animals for some portion of their protein. Even in Costa Rica, where fruit and other plant food sources are so abundant, the consensus among homesteaders I've talked with is that a pure fruitarian diet just doesn't work for humans. I have also met a surprising number of homesteaders who, like me, had been vegetarians for many years but were now raising rabbits, chickens, goats, and cows for protein. Why? Because growing animal products is easier.

Meat Makes Sense

There are three main reasons why animal food is easier to produce than plants. The first is the workload. Animals are just less work than annual gardens. As I described in Chapter 3, the chore of keeping chickens is easily manageable with automatic waterers, automatic feeders, and electric fencing. They water and feed themselves, and with access to the coop, run, and yard, the chickens will naturally move to a sunny spot if they are cold or to a shady spot if they are hot.

Your vegetables can't do that. You can put your watering system on a timer, but you'll still need to monitor it closely to adapt to rain patterns. You'll need to arrange cover to protect your plants from frosts and freezes, and you'll sometimes need to arrange shading. Feeding your garden means manually applying compost and fertilizers. None of this work is too much, but it still is more than what is needed for the animals.

The second reason is fertilizer. Nitrogen is one of the most essential elements for plants, and it just so happens that the form of nitrogen in animal waste is precisely the form plants want the most. Creating fertilizer by composting animal waste is faster than making compost from plants. It also takes much less space—you don't have to grow a bunch of plants simply to make compost from them. In fact, many vegetarians keep animals just for the fertilizer. Stacey Murphy of Grow Your Own Vegetables is one of many examples. Murphy is a vegetarian, but she keeps rabbits for their fertilizer, and she notices a big difference in vegetable production when she adds rabbit pellets to her garden.

The third reason is simply calories. You can produce far more calories and nutritional density with animals—and you can do it in a much smaller space than you would need if you did it solely with plants. In two growing seasons (the average time in a year that most gardeners will be able to grow across the United States), a beginner gardener can produce approximately 50,000 to 70,000 calories. A backyard flock of six laying hens, which requires about the same space, provides 94,500 calories. A home rabbitry with one buck and three breeding does, which also takes approximately the same amount of space, can produce 235,000 calories.

I don't want to discourage anyone who wants to remain purely vegetarian. But you should know that you will have to put in more time and a lot more work than those who produce animal products.

The Rhythm of Life and Death

When you buy your food from a grocery store, it's easy to forget the real relationship that humans have with our food. We live by taking the life of other things. Even an herbivore, like a rabbit, takes life from a plant to sustain itself. And when we die, the energy within our bodies eventually goes back to the plants, should we let them complete the cycle. (I'm glad to see the fledgling movement toward green burials that has started in the United States.)

What matters most is not the fact that an animal dies. That's inevitable. What matters most is how it lived and how it was honored at the end. The modern food production system treats animals worse than prisoners. It's a horrible, cruel system. The animals have no dignity or joy. Instead, they have only stress, pain, and fear, from birth until death. When you eat those products, you are taking those negative feelings into your body. But when you raise an animal with love and then end its life with honor and thankfulness, you create an honest connection to the cycle of life.

Some people are concerned that witnessing or taking part in the butchering process will traumatize children (or adults). I think this is a misconception—an irrational fear—that comes out of our unnatural separation from food production. Processing small game used to be a common skill among young and old alike. Years ago, when momma told the kids, "Get me a chicken," what she meant was go to the coop, butcher a bird, and bring her the processed bird, ready for her to cook.

Both my son, Ryan, and my daughter, Kimber, grew up raising and caring for animals. For many years, our family would raise a flock of meat chickens. It was a 3-month project that would give us free-range organic chicken all year long, plus enough extra to share with friends and family. The day-old baby chicks would arrive at the post office, and within a few months, we would raise the birds to size. At the end, in batches over two or three weekends, we would process them all. I was often surprised by how many of our kids' friends wanted to help during the processing weekends to learn how to do it.

Should you name your meat animals? It's common practice not to name them because your relationship is a bit different and usually much shorter than with your laying flock. But Kimber especially loves animals, and she always named them. When she was younger, she used to take the baby rabbits onto the trampoline to teach them how to jump. I didn't have the heart to tell her it wasn't necessary to teach baby rabbits how to jump, but the baby bunnies didn't seem to mind.

She's been there to welcome new lives into the world, and she's been there to witness their passing, whether that was from old age, disease, or a predator. And, yes, most of the time, we are the predators in that relationship. We are raising these animals for food, and Kimber has taken part in that. Like the children who would help us, Kimber was fascinated by the process. During the butchering, she wanted to learn the names and functions of all the organs. It's funny how kids will sometimes show you their future path. Kimber is in college now, studying to become a veterinarian. I know she'll be great because she loves animals, but she doesn't have the squeamishness some of her classmates display.

Why Rabbits?

Rabbits are the third part of the three-part Grow System for producing at least half of your own food in a backyard-sized space. With a 100-square-foot garden, a flock of six laying hens, and a home rabbitry, you can produce about 365,000 calories in a year in a backyard. That's about half of the calorie requirements, and most of the mineral and vitamin needs, for an adult human. Rabbits are also vital for cycling nutrients in your food production system, which increases the overall fertility and vibrancy of not only your yard but also your life.

Rabbits are far and away the best source of high-quality meat for a backyard system. They're quiet, easy to raise, and don't require a lot of space. And they are prolific—they breed like . . . rabbits. Three does and one buck can have 75 baby rabbits a year. That's about 1.5 rabbits a week for the dinner table and approximately half the protein requirements for a family of four.

What's more, they're herbivores, which makes them more cost-effective to feed. Animals like chickens and pigs are omnivores who like to eat a lot of the same things we do, which makes them direct competition for food sources. Omnivores' food is more expensive. On the other hand, rabbits will happily live off the kind of stuff most people would put out with the trash, like landscape trimmings, grass clippings, tree bark, and weeds.

Also, rabbit meat is a very tasty and versatile meat. It can be baked, roasted, grilled, stewed, slow-cooked, or used just about any other way you would cook chicken. In fact, one of the best ways to start using rabbit is to substitute it in any of your favorite chicken recipes. (Sometimes if I've forgotten to tell dinner guests I've served them rabbit, they just assume it's chicken.) I've used rabbit in stir-fries, sandwiches, enchiladas, and much more.

what's eating my garden?

Contrary to the cartoons, a rabbit is much more likely to eat your carrot tops than the carrot roots. Rabbits love to forage on fresh greens in the spring, summer, and fall. In the winter, they eat bark and twigs. Some people like to wrap the trunks of their young fruit trees in winter to protect them from the naughty nibblers.

The Basic Recipe
for a Backyard Rabbitry

Ingredients
3 breeding does

1 buck

Housing

Watering system

Feed

breeding like rabbits

Did you know that rabbits live on every continent except Antarctica? These energetic animals have hippity-hopped their way across the entire planet, breeding as they went. But not all rabbits raise their young in burrows, like you see in children's books. Instead of digging holes, some rabbits prefer to make small ground nests.

Bunny Breeds

As with chickens, a rabbit's anatomy is the first overall consideration for choosing the right rabbits for your region. When I was homesteading in Texas, which is primarily a hot place, I had rabbits that were small with short fur. I especially liked the Rex breed, which has very short fur and tends to be on the small side, because rabbits can die from heatstroke and don't breed well during the summer. I recently learned from Dr. Steven D. Lukefahr, coauthor of one of my favorite go-to reference books, *Rabbit Production*, that Texas A&M is researching a way to breed furless or "naked" rabbits. We'll see if that comes to pass, but right now almost all breeds handle the cold much better than the heat.

The two most common backyard meat breeds are Californians and New Zealands. Both do well almost everywhere. However, when you are just starting out, I suggest you get mixed-breed rabbits like you'll find on craigslist. They will likely be different colored or have distinct markings so you can easily identify who is who, they cost less than purebreds, and mixed breeds tend to be more resilient.

Be certain the buck has a different bloodline from the does. Inbreeding is never good in any species. The offspring are weaker and prone to degenerative diseases.

And as with the chickens, visiting the seller's rabbitry can tell you volumes about the rabbits' quality. Plus, you'll have a new friend and resource for questions.

When you get skilled in raising both chickens and rabbits, I encourage you to become a champion for a rare breed or two. Because homesteading has dropped by the wayside for the past few generations, many useful livestock breeds have gone extinct. Similar to the heirloom varieties of fruits and vegetables, most breeds were developed by people like you and me for the particular needs of the families who were producing their own food. By contrast, most of our modern livestock breeding has been focused on the needs of large-scale commercial agriculture. Those animals are of little use in family-scale food production. I talk more about this in Chapter 11, but for now, know you can make a massive difference to your family and your community for generations to come by helping reestablish or develop useful breeds of backyard rabbits.

Hutches

As with chickens, the absolute best place for your rabbits to live is under a big deciduous tree. Keeping your rabbits cool is going to be a much bigger challenge than keeping them warm, and nothing is so soothing in the summertime as the deep shade under a big tree. And just like the chickens, the tree will love the companionship and extra fertilization the rabbits will give it.

If you don't have free space under a big tree, a protected area such as under a carport, next to the house, or in a shed is also good.

You will want a separate hutch for each of your four breeders, the buck and three does. The hutches should have at least 12 square feet of space per rabbit. You can either build individual hutches or combine them together into a complex. In Texas, I built a four-hutch complex that is 2.5 feet wide by 20 feet long and takes up only 50 square feet.

You'll also need small movable pens known as "rabbit tractors" to raise the babies. The tractors are also useful as exercise pens. You can use them to allow the buck and does to get out of the hutches from time to time. (More on rabbit tractors in the next section.)

Like the chicken coop, these structures are easy to build over a few weekends. I have provided a link for a free downloadable set of building plans for both the hutches and tractors in the resources section at the end of this chapter. The plans include step-by-step directions, 3D drawings, a parts list, and a tools list.

When you assemble your system, be sure to elevate the hutches off the ground. This helps protect them from predators, and it also puts them at a convenient height for you to access them.

Here is a list of the characteristics of an ideal backyard rabbit hutch:

- 12 square feet per rabbit

- Interior should be at least 24 inches tall (Rabbits like to stand up on their hind legs.)

- It should be elevated off the ground

- Ease of access for cleaning up/removal of the rabbit pellets with large, easy-to-open doors

- 1×2-inch wire for the sides and top

- 1½×1-inch wire mesh for the floor and bottom 4 inches of the sides (This relieves pressure on the rabbits' feet and keeps baby rabbits from accidently falling out.)

- Removable nest boxes 12 inches wide × 12 inches tall × 18 inches long for each doe, with doors wide enough to allow easy entry for the nesting box

- Secure, raccoon-proof latches

- Roof with large overhang on all sides

- A safe place for the rabbits to hide: one corner with three solid sides and a top

- Removable panels for the sides and back to seasonally adjust for protection from the cold and winds

- Watering system with redundant nipples for each hutch

- Gravity-fed feeders (I like the ones with the mesh bottoms.)

- A flat piece of solid board inside each hutch for the rabbits to lie or sit on (This also relieves stress on the rabbits' feet.)

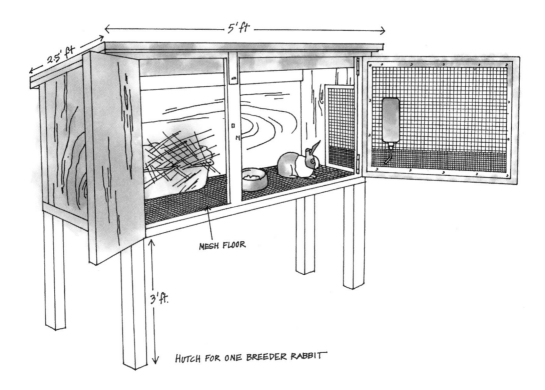

5' ft

2.5' ft

MESH FLOOR

3' ft.

HUTCH FOR ONE BREEDER RABBIT

Backyard Rabbit Tractors

Rabbit tractors are movable pens you'll put the weaned bunnies into to let them grow out to full size. (And when you aren't using them to raise babies, they also make excellent exercise pens for the breeder rabbits who live in the hutches—kind of like a fun vacation for them.) The name is somewhat misleading, though. Contrary to what it implies, you will be the one doing all the pulling. Every day, you will move the tractors the length of each tractor to give the bunnies access to fresh grass. Grass is a natural and preferred food for rabbits, and as a bonus, it saves you money on their feed bill.

I have experimented with all kinds of tractor designs. What I like best is a 3-foot-wide by 6-foot-long by 2-foot-tall tractor made from mostly 2×2-inch wood. This size is very lightweight and easy to move around the yard by women or children. But you can experiment with different sizes. I once build a tractor that was 5 feet wide by 8 feet long by 4 feet tall, purposefully making it big enough that I could sit inside. At the time, I was experimenting with keeping the breeding stock in tractors, and I became very connected with a red doe named Mae Ren. (The name Mae Ren was one in a series of Japanese names Kimber gave the rabbits while she was in her anime phase.) Mae Ren was initially very shy. Every morning I did my meditation in the tractor without trying to touch her or engage her at all. After a while, she became so comfortable with me that she would hop into my lap and meditate with me. I miss her now and still consider her a good friend.

Smaller, lightweight tractors are much more practical, less expensive, and easier to build and move. I recommend three rabbit tractors, for a total of only 54 square feet.

Here are the characteristics of the ideal backyard rabbit tractor:

- 3 feet wide × 6 feet long × 2 feet tall

- Lightweight—mostly 2×2-inch construction boards

- 2×4-inch frame on the bottom for strength

- The entire solid roof should have a hinged opening to allow for easy access to the whole tractor

- Raccoon-proof latches

- 1×1-inch wire mesh fencing on all sides

- 2×4-inch wire mesh fencing on the bottom

- $\frac{1}{3}$ of the tractor should have walls that form a protected area

- Large gravity-fed feeder (I like the ones with the mesh bottoms.)

- At least two sources of water, either bottles or a gravity-fed bucket and nipples arrangement

- Rope handles on each end for pulling

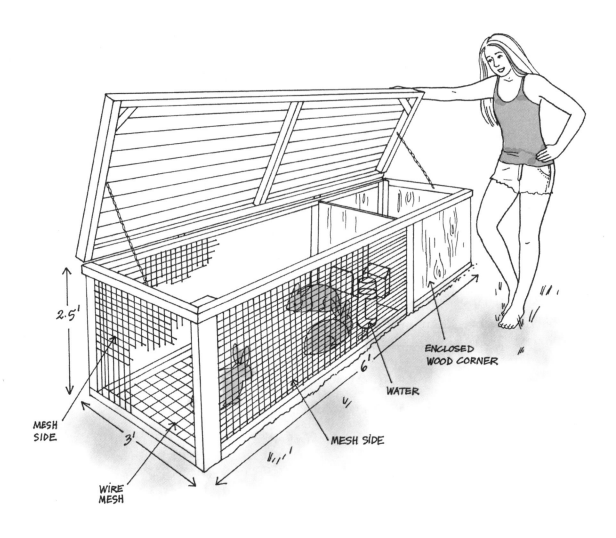

To those of you who are serious builders, the lightweight construction of mostly 2×2 may seem flimsy. And yes, it is flimsy. But it is also astonishing how long these rabbit tractors last. Yes, sometimes you do have to replace some boards, but all the other components will wear well and can be reused for many, many years—decades even. I promise you that a super-durable tractor will weigh too much and you won't want to use it.

It is best if you move the tractors to fresh grass every day. Rabbit tractors are the ultimate "weed and feed" system. What I found delightful, when putting the tractors in the yard for the first time, was the trail of beautiful green left in their wake. After a while, you'll be building up so much fertilizer in your lawn that the difference won't be as noticeable. But that first pass through is amazing.

Some people have concerns that the fencing on the bottom might accidentally break a bunny's leg as you're moving it. Just keep the tractor low to the ground and go slow as you pull. The rabbits quickly learn and adapt. The bottom fencing is important because it allows the grass to come through but keeps the rabbits from digging out (and they love digging!). It also keeps predators from digging in from underneath.

10 minutes of daily tasks

On most days, your rabbitry will practically run itself. You can keep it going with a commitment of less than 10 minutes per day to perform the following tasks:

Check water and feed levels

Check nesting boxes and breeding schedule

Move the rabbit tractors

Food

In the beginning, I recommend you make it easy on yourself and buy high-quality rabbit food. Rabbits need high-quality pellets, hay, and perhaps something to chew on. The pellets should contain all the minerals and a bulk of the nutrition the rabbits need. Definitely check the label because many commercial rabbit pellets contain genetically modified ingredients, which you want to avoid. The hay is roughage for the rabbits, which they also need. You can toss in a small piece of wood, maybe 6 or 8 inches long, for the rabbits to chew on. A small piece of firewood, a piece of untreated 2×4 pine, sticks, and fresh branches also are good things for rabbits to chew on. A rabbit's teeth are always growing, and they need to gnaw and chew on tough, woody materials to keep their teeth worn down and in check.

One important note: your does need a lot of high-quality food when they are pregnant and nursing, but you don't want to let them get fat. If you can't feel a doe's ribs anymore and she won't breed, it's time to cut back a little.

It is fairly easy to produce at least half of your rabbits' diets from garden weeds, yard clippings, and landscape trimmings. It's entirely doable, but it's probably not something most beginners want to jump into. For that reason, I recommend you start out buying commercial feed. It has a balance of nutrients your rabbits need, it's easy to pour into a gravity feeder, and it's one less thing to think about while you're gaining confidence raising rabbits.

Pellets

On the other end of this system—literally—is poop. Believe it or not, this "waste" is actually a precious resource. Rabbit manure provides excellent fertilizer for your garden. It's small, has little odor, and is packaged in a convenient pellet form for easy distribution.

Rabbit pellets are considered "cold" manure, meaning you can put them directly around the base of your plants. By contrast, chicken manure is "hot" and needs to be composted before applying to your garden. So sprinkling a few "handfuls" (no, you don't have to actually use your hands) of rabbit pellets around your garden makes your plants very happy. The pellets feed the garden, and the garden can supply extra greens for the rabbits. Don't you just love a complementary system?

Many people set up a worm composting bin underneath their rabbit hutches. The worms love the manure, and worm castings are an even more amazing fertilizer than the pellets alone. In fact, I know of many small commercial rabbitries that are not commercially viable selling rabbits, meat, and fur. Instead, what makes them profitable is the additional revenue they take in from worms and worm castings grown in the rabbits' pellets.

Breeding

Rabbits need to be at least 6 months old before you can breed them. Unlike most other mammals, rabbits can be bred at any time of year. It is difficult to get them to breed in extreme heat. (No one wants to be pregnant in a Texas summer.) Also, if the buck or the doe is too fat, they will not be as likely to breed.

A biological quirk of rabbits is that they don't ovulate until after they've been bred. That makes rabbits an ideal animal for novice breeders. You don't have to wait for a certain time or watch for specific indicators. You've just got to put them in a room together and let nature take its course.

However, there are a few things you can do to help things move along smoothly. First, always bring the doe to the buck's cage. Does are highly territorial and may see the buck's arrival as a threat. When the doe and buck are together, they may sniff each other or chase each other around for a while. The buck may stomp. You will hear them make a lot of noises you've never associated with rabbits before. All of this is natural.

If the doe is inclined to mate, she will lie down with her backside offered up to the buck. If she's not impressed, or just not in the mood, she may sit up, pressing her back end down and hiding it altogether. Or the chasing around the cage won't stop. If either one acts aggressively toward the other, you should remove the doe from the pen. Don't leave them stuck with each other, and never leave them alone. Unhappy rabbits are capable of maiming or killing one another.

Hopefully, everything will go smoothly. The buck will mount the doe, and he may bite her neck to keep his position. That's normal, and he's not really hurting her. He'll get to work right away, and when he's done, you'll know it. It happens really quickly. He often gives a little yelp and then he will fall, quite dramatically, on his side. It's probably the funniest thing you'll see all day. It is very clear *he* had a good time. You can allow the buck to go at it two or maybe three times in a session, but then take away the doe for a while to let him rest. I suggest bringing the doe for another visit within a couple of hours. Remember that rabbits ovulate after mating. This will give the egg some extra time to get into position and meet the sperm.

If nothing happens within 5 minutes, remove the doe and try again later.

In your journal or record-keeping system (more on that coming up), note the name of the doe, the date she was bred, and with whom. (You only have one buck right now, but you'll be surprised how useful this info can be later.)

It's important to keep records so you can put a nesting box in her hutch in approximately 28 days from the breeding. You can either make nesting boxes or buy them. The box should be mostly closed and approximately 12 inches wide by 12 inches tall by 18 inches long. That is plenty of room for most average-sized meat-breed rabbits. If you've never done any carpentry before, making a nest box is the perfect beginner project. Just be sure the finished nest box will fit through the hutch door.

You can reuse a nesting box. Be sure to clean it first by letting it sit out in the sun for a few hours. Sunlight is a great sanitizer.

In 28 days, provide the doe with her nesting box, along with straw, hay, or other soft, dry materials to pad it. The doe will make a nest in the box by organizing the materials you gave her and pulling her own fur to make it super comfy.

After you've placed the nesting box in the doe's hutch, don't move it. And unless you usually handle your doe a lot, don't bother her either. She is pregnant, after all, and keeping her stress levels down is going to help her develop healthy babies.

About 31 days after the breeding, you'll find a litter of between 2 and 14 adorable little baby rabbits, or kits; about 8 is average. You really don't have to do much here. Just ooh and aah a little, take a picture, and have your kids peek in. But mostly give the mother privacy.

As you check in on her, you may notice the momma rabbit seems like she's not giving enough attention to her little ones. Don't worry. Rabbits are not doting or super attentive. This is rooted in their practical reality; rabbits know they're prey animals, so by "ignoring" her babies, the doe is not drawing attention to them. She may feed them only once or twice a day, and you probably won't ever see her doing it.

Death is a regular visitor on farms and homesteads, and if you raise animals, sooner or later you're going to have to deal with a dead one. It's not uncommon for one or more of the litter to be stillborn, and sometimes the runt of the litter isn't viable enough to make it.

On your daily checks, peek in to see that everyone is alive. The mother will often bury the dead one in a corner of the nest box away from the others, so gently feel around for that. Remove any dead rabbits as soon as possible to prevent bacteria from growing. It's not pleasant, but it's a reality you'll need to be prepared for. My farm dogs often accompany me during my morning rabbit chores in the hope of getting a stillborn baby rabbit snack.

Theoretically, you could breed your doe again, almost right away. The doe is fully capable of nursing her young and growing a new litter at the same time. Rabbit numbers can really go wild when they're motivated. But it's not easy on them, and I don't recommend it. Very aggressive breeders might try for six and a half litters per year, but a healthier amount is four or five per year. This gives the doe some time to rest, recover, and replenish her reserves. I wait at least a month before rebreeding. Also, remember that in some climates, especially extremely hot ones, you won't be able to breed throughout the entire year. In Texas, I was happy with four litters per year but usually got three.

Young rabbits are fully able to start feeding themselves by 4 weeks old, but nursing helps them put on healthy weight in a hurry. Leaving them with the doe a bit longer helps you grow larger rabbits faster. The best time to start weaning is around 6 weeks old.

When you move the youngsters out to the tractor, put mom out there with them for a few days to a week and then return her to her hutch. She will enjoy being out on the grass, and her being with them will help with the transition. Removing her actually mimics what happens in nature: in the wild, the mother rabbit will leave to go dig another burrow and let the young fend for themselves.

Record-Keeping

I know it might seem like you can keep this all in your head. It's just three does, right? But trust me. After a while, everything starts running together. Do yourself a *huge* favor and keep records. I'll lay out the simplest method here to get you started.

First, create tags for each of your breeders (the buck and the three does) and for the litters. These tags will be attached to the hutches and tractors with carabiners or twist ties to identify the rabbits, or the rabbits' parents. I highly recommend you get the tags laminated or otherwise waterproofed. Using a waterproof Sharpie on laminated card works great. When you need to reuse a tag, you can remove the writing with rubbing alcohol.

Here is the basic data you want on your tags for the breeders:

Name

Hutch number

Date of birth

Color/markings

Bred date

Nesting box date

Weaned date

Here is the basic data you want on your tags for each litter:

Litter ID

Number of kits

Doe name

Buck name

Kindled date

Weaned date

Butchered date

In addition to the tags, you'll want to keep a log of the breeding. Trust me, you really do want to do this. I'm a bit old-fashioned and keep it all on a printed Excel spreadsheet on a clipboard. I have a big repurposed mailbox next to my rabbitry that holds my clipboard along with miscellaneous hand tools and supplies. Using an old mailbox is a great way to keep it all dry.

You want to have one page per doe. Here is the basic info and an example to get you started. There is a lot more data you could keep, but this is a great starting point.

Doe name

Color

Date of birth

Doe Name: **SUNNY**
Color/markings: **white/tan markings**
DOB: **Jan. 2018 (est.)**

Buck name	Bred date	Nest box date	Expected kindle date	Actual kindle date	Date Live	Dead	Re-breed date	Wean date	Butcher date
Rumple	2/4/2019	3/4/2019	3/7/2019	3/6/2019	8	0	tbd	4/16/2019	7/13/2019
Rumple									
Rumple	9/2/2019	9/30/2019	10/3/2019	10/4/2019	9	1	11/14/2019	11/18/2019	3/2/2020
Rumple	11/14/2019	12/12/2019	12/15/2019	12/17/2019	8	0	1/15/2020	1/31/2020	5/18/2020
Rumple	1/15/2020	2/12/2020	2/13/2020	2/13/2020	8	0	3/14/2020	3/30/2020	6/27/2020

Processing Your Rabbits

Many people start out thinking they can't do something like this, but so often they're surprised at how humane and respectful the process can be. I've had many vegetarians watch and later tell me, "That was done so lovingly. Even though I don't eat meat, if I ever change my mind, that's how I'd want it to be handled."

I've taught thousands of people how to do this, and it's always easier than they think. A professional can do it in about 3 minutes, but from setup to cleanup, it takes me about 15 to 20 minutes.

The optimal feed-to-weight range for a rabbit is at around 2 to 3 months. I usually procrastinate and end up waiting a bit longer, until they're around 4 to 5 months. This will yield about a 6-pound rabbit. The meat-to-carcass ratio for rabbits is 60 percent, so a 6-pound rabbit has about 3.5 pounds of meat.

I suggest you remove the food from the rabbit's trailer 12 to 24 hours before you process it so you won't have to deal with a full intestinal tract. This isn't a necessity, but it does make things a little easier.

Collect your tools. You'll want a broom, a sharp knife, butcher paper, and a cutting board. Tin snips are helpful but not necessary. I have a crude kitchen and a sink with running water in the barn I use, but you can do this with a hose or a 5-gallon bucket of water.

Before you can process a rabbit, it has to die. This is the hardest part for people. I don't enjoy it either. Actually, that is why my rabbits tend to be a lot bigger than the optimal feed-to-weight timing—I tend to procrastinate on this chore. The key is to do it as quickly and painlessly for the rabbit as possible. Place the rabbit on the floor, and lay a broom handle across its neck. Stand on the broom handle, with one foot on either side of the rabbit. Grab the rabbit's back feet, and pull up with a hard, fast motion. You should feel a crack as the neck breaks.

Death isn't always instant, but it will come very quickly. A certain amount of twitching is common either way. That has to do with the sudden damage to the rabbit's nervous system, rather than any actual pain.

It is entirely appropriate to say any words of thanks or prayers at this point. Sing a song. Cry if you feel like it. It's okay. Tears can honor the rabbit, too. I always offer prayers and sing a song of compassion.

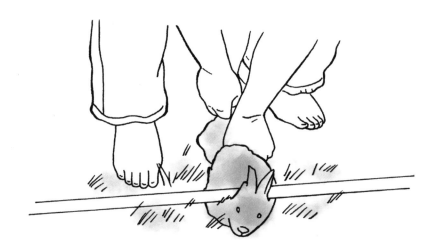

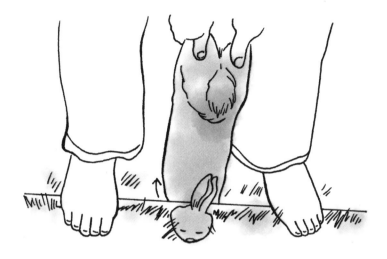

After you've passed this hurdle, you can move on to the processing. First, you'll want to wet the rabbit's fur. It is not entirely necessary, but it helps keep stray hairs from getting into the meat. Next, use your knife to cut the skin in a circle around the rabbit's hocks, or back feet.

Cutting through fur will dull your knife quickly, so as soon as you have an opening, stick your knife through and cut from underneath. After you've gotten all the way around both hocks, go up the legs until you have enough skin to get a good grip. Hold the foot in one hand, and pull the skin with the other. In effect, it's a bit like pulling off a sweater. When you get to the front feet, you can either pull until the skin tears or cut it away with your knife.

If you want to tan the skin, avoid using the knife as much as possible, except to cut off the tail. Otherwise, the knife can be used to help you get past any difficult spots.

Keep pulling until you reach the rabbit's head. Cut the skin here, and set it aside. If you aren't going to tan the skin, it makes good dog food, hair and all. The skin contains a lot of good nutrition, and your dogs will poop out the undigested fur.

Next, cut off the rabbit's head. This will be easier because you've already broken the neck.

This is a good time to get out a bag for any of the parts you aren't going to use, like the feet, head, and intestines. These parts could be eaten by humans, but I use them for dog food. If you're working by a sink or a hose, this is also a good time to wash off the rabbit to remove any dirt or stray hairs.

If you're using tin snips, cut through the bone and remove the rabbit's feet. If you're using a knife, cut through the ligaments around the foot joint and then twist and bend the rabbit's foot to snap it off.

Around this time, it's not uncommon to notice twitching muscles. Don't panic! The rabbit is completely dead, and it's not feeling anything. I promise. Muscle spasms might be a little unsettling, but they're totally normal.

Lay the rabbit on its back, and cut up from the bottom of the belly to the ribs. Be careful not to cut too deep, or you'll puncture the intestines. One way to prevent this is to start with a small hole, just large enough to get two fingers into. Use your fingers to hold the wall of the belly up, away from the organs. Insert the knife, with the cutting edge facing up, and carefully work your way forward.

Now that the organs are exposed, take a look at them and see if you can identify them. Check that the organs look healthy, too. This won't be obvious at first, but with practice, it will become clearer. Look for strange colors, worms, or anything odd and out of place. There rarely are problems with rabbits, so don't stress about this, but do start learning.

You can scoop out the organs, mostly by hand, but use the knife if needed. Save the heart, kidneys, and liver. We'll deal with those in a moment. Some native people ate the intestines, and some homesteaders use them for sausage casings, but I primarily reserve those for the dogs to eat.

Rinse the rabbit off again, using your hand to clear out any remnants in the organ cavity. Now you've got a whole rabbit ready for roasting, or you can quarter it or cut it into smaller, conveniently sized pieces. It's now ready for cooking, refrigerating, or freezing.

who else eats rabbit?

For many Americans, rabbit is not a "normal" meat. Many people would rather stick to chicken, beef, pork, and fish. But rabbit is a favorite, or even gourmet, food in many places around the world. The top rabbit-meat-consuming countries in the world are China, Italy, the Democratic People's Republic of Korea, Egypt, and Spain.

The Zen of Rabbit Processing

Processing rabbits is challenging emotionally. Butchering *should* challenge everyone emotionally. In fact, many small farmers rotate out this chore because if you aren't emotionally engaged, if you've done it so much you can't feel anything, then you've lost touch with something vital and you should not be doing the work.

Once I spent several hours before processing a rabbit in deep meditation. I contemplated how in this reality in which we live, life is based on death. I focused on how my own body is only here for a fleeting moment and how life is a continual process of eating, excreting, growing, and dying. That is true for every microbe, every plant, and every creature. I felt fluid and graceful as I removed the older doe from her hutch. I spoke to her gently and told her what I was going to do, that she would be going on another adventure soon. I let her know how much I appreciated her body. She was so peaceful in my arms as I carried her up to the barn. As I gently put her on the floor, she was completely relaxed, and to my astonishment, she laid out her neck. I put the broomstick across her and called my internal strength I needed to perform the quick motion that would kill her. And then I saw her body completely relax without the slightest twitch or twitter. Normally there are some convulsions when a body dies, but she left hers in complete peace.

I believe we were both conscious of, and accepting of, what I was doing. Since then, I've read about others who have had that experience, too. It only happened for me that one time, maybe because I haven't had time since to meditate before processing. But that one experience has me wondering if there are other ways we could be working with our livestock.

Don't Throw Out the Best Parts

The muscle isn't the only part of the rabbit you can eat. These days so many of us get our meat at the grocery store, where it has already been processed and butchered, and we've forgotten how to use the whole animal.

The organs contain a huge amount of nutrition, particularly the heart, liver, and kidneys. Organ meats are the most nutritionally dense superfoods you can produce in your backyard. Many people of my age and older remember when eating liver once a week was a required meal. Even though I complained about liver as a kid, now I understand why moms have always served this traditional food. Liver not only contains high-quality protein, but it's also nature's most abundant source of vitamin A, it contains all the B vitamins, and it's full of a highly usable form of iron. Several trace elements, such as copper, zinc, chromium, and coenzyme Q10 (CoQ10), are also found in the liver. Rich nutrition like this is the main key to building vibrant health! One easy way to reintroduce these precious foods into your diet is to dice the organ meats and add them to chilis or stews. Or make a liver pâté and eat it with crackers.

Please do not eat the organs from commercially farmed animals. They've absorbed and concentrated many toxins from the system they were raised in. But the organ meats from your rabbits will be clean, healthy, and deeply nutritious. You know exactly what your animals ate, and you can be assured it was clean. Our ancestors highly revered the organ meats because they knew their nutritional value. In the past, these were the foods often reserved for pregnant women, elders, leaders, and royalty—that's how special they are.

Don't throw out the bones! At first, my family was a little bit leery of bone broths, but we all watched a PBS special in which Julia Child made bone broths and explained how these special liquids are the secret essence of great gourmet dishes. Bone broth is rich in magnesium, zinc, potassium, and collagen. My mom always had a stockpot of broth going on the back of the stove. As a young woman, I often was mystified why my soups tasted so watery and flat—nothing like Mom's. It wasn't until I started making bone broths that I understood and was able to make truly delicious soups and stews.

If you are squeamish about processing your own meat, believe me, I completely understand. Check around. I am willing to bet that someone you know who loves hunting or fishing knows how to process game. You can also ask at your local farmers market about local animal processors. Some farmers do it themselves and might be willing to do a batch for you during one of their usual runs. Other farmers contract out the work to small processing centers. Either way, you are likely to find someone or a business that can take care of it for you.

chapter summary

- Rabbits are an ideal animal for backyard meat production.

- Pellets are a secret bonus to raising rabbits.

- Three does and one buck can produce 75 rabbits a year. That's around 1.5 rabbits a week for the dinner table, and approximately half the protein requirements for a family of four.

- Processing rabbits isn't fun, but it can be done humanely and with gratitude.

- For food purposes, rabbit meat can be treated like chicken.

- Organ meats are the most nutrient-dense foods you can produce at home. You are what you eat.

additional resources

For more information on raising rabbits, check out these websites:
- www.BackyardRabbitHutchPlans.com. A free set of step-by-step plans for building the rabbit hutch and tractors described in this chapter, including variations for different climates.

- www.GrowYourOwnGroceries.com. Section 4 of this 10-part video shows how I process rabbits. And because people have asked me the origin of the song I sing to honor the animal's life, I'll tell you now—it's a badly done rendition of a song of compassion I heard the Dalai Lama sing. And when I say "badly done," I mean it. But the spirit and intent come through.

- www.ColonyRabbits.com. A video documenting my experimental system of raising rabbits in a semi-free-range colony. This is part of my ongoing work to find even more honorable ways to raise rabbits.

- www.MeatChickens.com. Each year my family and I raise a flock of meat chickens as a part of our food supply. One year I decided to get out a camera and film the process . . . and everything went wrong. We still managed to have a freezer full of meat, though. Join and watch over my shoulder as I go through that crazy summer, laugh a lot, and learn what not to do.

chapter 5

the soil: compost and other secrets to a green thumb

I had not realized the magnitude of the transformation I had undergone until I saw Janet.

Janet Snyder was wearing boots, thick socks, thermal underlayers, a heavy coat, gloves, scarf, and a hat. We were in central Idaho attending a primitive skills gathering known as Rabbit Stick.

A primitive skills gathering is where people come together to learn and exchange skills from the Paleolithic era. My daughter and I used to go every year to play "cave-women" for the week, learning how to tan deerskins using the brains of the animal, making fire by friction, digging clay from the earth for pottery, navigating by the stars, foraging for wild edibles, and making traps and snares. The event happens in late September each year, so it is typical for the grass outside our tent to be crunchy with frost.

Affectionately known as "Camp Mom," Janet offered me a mug of coffee early one morning that had a geyser of steam coming from it. While we caught up, I could not stop staring at her, noticing the difference between us. Or more accurately, the difference in myself.

I grew up in South Florida and had zero tolerance for cold weather. Snow was an imaginary concept I saw only on Christmas cards. If the temperature dropped below 70 degrees Fahrenheit, I reached for a sweater. When I attended the University of Florida, it was always easy to spot the northern kids who still sported shorts and T-shirts when the temps dipped slightly, while us southerners were bundled from head to toe. For most of my life since then, I had always managed to live in warm or hot climates.

But here I was, engaging in morning chitchat with Janet, comfortably accepting the mug of coffee with my bare hands while standing there in my bare feet, jeans, shirt, a light jacket, and a beanie.

Sure, I felt the cold, but I wasn't uncomfortable.

How had this transformation happened? Just a few days prior I had left my home in Texas, where it was pushing close to 100 degrees Fahrenheit. And yet, here in this freezing world, I was fine.

I was dumbstruck. How had I gained this amazing ability? It took me a while to connect the dots. The answer will probably surprise you, too. My high tolerance to both cold and heat came from my garden soil.

Early Adventures in Poor Soils

When I first decided to start growing food, I admittedly didn't know a lot. I definitely didn't understand how important soil is. I thought soil was just "dirt." It's only there to hold the plants, right? We stand on it. Grass grows in it. It's dusty when it's dry and muddy when it's wet. It's something to be cleaned up when it gets into the house. Dirt. I thought of it like an inanimate object, when I thought about it at all. Just a background element of life.

It wasn't until I first tried to grow broccoli that I started to see what I was missing. I bought a cute little packet of seeds with a picture of big, beautiful, green broccoli heads on the front. The instructions on the packet couldn't be simpler: 1) Plant seeds. 2) Water seeds. 3) Harvest broccoli. So easy!

As I planted the seeds, I started daydreaming about what I would have to do to fit all the broccoli in my refrigerator when harvest day came. As it turned out, that wasn't the problem I was going to face. When the broccoli came up spindly and pale, my confidence was shaken a little. They stayed the same shape, stubbornly refused to get any bigger, and continued to fade a little each day.

Then, one night we had a light cold snap. I went out the next day to check on my broccoli and found them fallen over and dead (as dead as the soil I was trying to grow them in). I groaned in frustration. What went wrong? Broccoli is a cool-weather plant. That cold spell shouldn't have affected them like this.

I decided to look for answers. I visited different farmers and gardeners in the area. My neighbor Brandon always had an amazing garden, so I dropped by to see how his broccoli was doing. When he led me back through the gate to his garden, my jaw dropped. His plants were so big and happy. His broccoli were huge and bursting with life. The cold hadn't bothered them one bit—if anything, they seemed extra perky. *This must be where they take the pictures for the seed packets*, I thought, because Brandon's broccoli was just like those photos—probably better.

"Brandon, how did you do this?!" I asked. I was ready for anything. Was it a secret planting technique? Was he buying a super-expensive, super-rare fish emulsion fertilizer, made from an endangered Tibetan cavefish? Was it a special variety of broccoli? Did he have to sacrifice a goat by the light of a full moon?

Brandon's answer wasn't nearly as exotic or mysterious as I imagined. His secret . . . was horseshit. Loads and loads of it. Brandon was gardening in 2 feet of composted manure.

Brandon is a farrier. He and his wife, Carrie, love horses and always keep several at their homestead. They give their animals the highest-quality feed, so the manure coming out of those horses is also of the highest quality and especially rich in minerals. It's no wonder Brandon's plants were so happy. They were the best-fed broccoli in the county.

Soil matters. I was growing my broccoli in an impoverished, sandy soil. It had next to no nutrients and retained water about as well as a fishing net. Brandon's soil was so stuffed with nutrients, those plants couldn't help but become paragons of broccoliness.

The Living Soil

Compost improves the texture of the soil, helping it retain moisture without becoming soggy and waterlogged. It also allows the roots to easily push through and grow wherever they want. And I've already mentioned the nutritional benefit for the plants, but I haven't mentioned the life it has.

Soil is alive. Well, my sandy soil wasn't . . . or maybe just barely. But Brandon's soil was filled with a variety of beneficial bacteria, fungi, burrowing bugs and worms, and a whole host of other microscopic life. They were all working and thriving together in a complex, beautiful web of activity. Worms and burrowing insects aerate the soil in addition to breaking down larger chunks. Bacteria also break down soil parts into usable products, but they fulfill another critical role, creating compounds the plants can absorb and use to be strong and healthy. The fungi act as messengers and nutrition transporters, carrying chemical signals and resources back and forth through the soil.

The soil in your garden is equivalent to your gut microbiome. Just as the microbes in your gut break down your food into usable nutrition that can be sent through your bloodstream to every part of your body, plants get their nutrition from a synergistic relationship with the microbes in the soil.

Through the magic of photosynthesis, plants use the energy of the sun to break down the carbon in carbon dioxide (CO_2) and hydration from water (H_2O) to make carbohydrates, specifically glucose ($C_6H_{12}O_6$). A by-product of the process is oxygen (O_2), which the plants don't need, but we do. The plant uses the glucose to make flowers, fruits, and other plant parts. We make use of those, too. Some of the glucose is sent down and excreted through the plant's roots to feed the surrounding bacteria, fungi, and other microbiology. In exchange for the glucose, the microbes break down the soil particles into usable elements to provide minerals the plant needs.

The microbiology in the soil effectively extends the roots of plants—sometimes for miles for older, established trees.

You and I are a part of a never-ending cycle of life that involves a complex web of mutually beneficial giving and receiving. The more you participate in the process, the healthier and happier you will become. The web is all around you, including down into the earth beneath your feet.

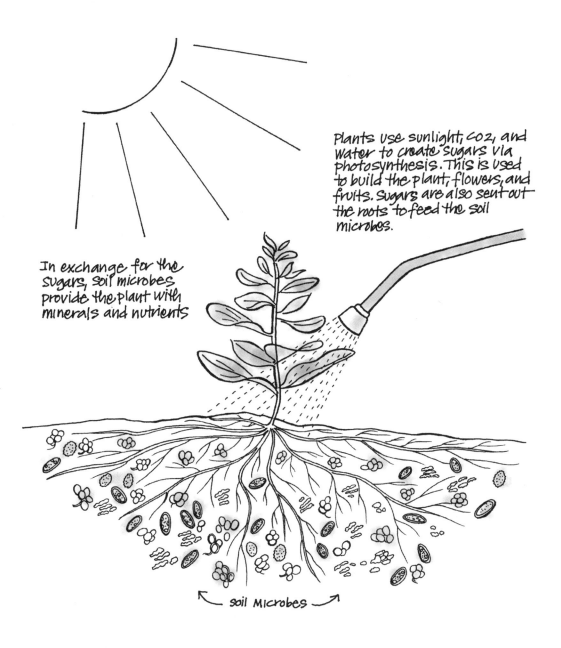

Plants use sunlight, CO2, and water to create sugars via photosynthesis. This is used to build the plant, flowers, and fruits. Sugars are also sent out the roots to feed the soil microbes.

In exchange for the sugars, soil microbes provide the plant with minerals and nutrients

← soil microbes →

Good soil—really good soil—is literally churning with life. You can cheat the system for a while with pesticides and chemical fertilizers, but chemical fertilizers don't support soil life, and pesticides kill off the soil's microbes and beneficial animal life. Over time, as the soil dies, the plants in it require more and more care and will never have the kind of health Brandon's plants had, naturally and effortlessly. It's kind of like eating sugar and junk food—it feels good in the short term but is a deadly, no-win game because it destroys your natural web of life.

If your soil isn't healthy, your plants won't be healthy. And if your plants aren't healthy, they can't pass on any health to you. Your health depends on the health of your soil.

Standing barefoot in the crisp Idaho morning, my hands warmed by a mug of coffee and my heart warmed by conversation with a good friend, is when I deeply understood the connection between the life and nutrition in my garden soil and my surprising new superpower of cold tolerance.

The foods we eat pass on their properties to us. On the one hand, this is quite obvious. Citrus fruits are high in vitamin C. When we eat them, they pass on that vitamin C to us. But this transference goes so much deeper than the nutrition label on the back of a product.

We Are Connected to Our Soil

Whenever you go outside, you experience the same environment as your local plants. You and they are facing the same environmental pressures. The plants make changes within their bodies to adapt to these pressures, and when we eat them, those changes get passed on to us.

After learning the importance of good soil from Brandon, the broccoli I grew enjoyed the cool weather and really thrived in it. Now, I realized, I did, too. And it doesn't just apply to cold weather. I no longer have the severe allergies that once plagued me, and a host of other health issues are just gone. High-quality nutrition is a universal part of all the world's healing practices, no matter what kind of disease or ailment you would like to heal.

You won't get that by eating foods from a grocery store. Those plants just don't have the same nutrition or vitality to give. Even if they did, they've been shipped hundreds of miles and lost a lot of their benefits. But the plants in your own backyard garden are as local, as fresh, and as nutritious as you could ever get.

That's the magic of homegrown foods. You're not just growing a garden and small livestock. You're growing your biggest primary assets: your health and resiliency.

As I touched on in Chapter 1, if you are just starting out, I recommend you buy the highest-quality soil you can afford for your garden. It will more than pay off in the long run. I'm a big fan of saving money when I can, but this is one of the last areas where I would try to pinch pennies because most of us just don't have very good soil in our backyards.

Our Disappearing Soil

When our country was founded, our ancestors knew the importance of good soil. They had to live off what they grew, and why not live where it is easiest to produce crops? Most of our major cities are places that were initially small areas settled because the soil there was good and water was close by. Historically, the price of land was determined not by how nice the house was but by the productivity of the soil.

Over the years, the cities grew and grew and became concreted over. Stripping off the topsoil is a part of the building process when suburbs are created. And most of the rural land now available would have never been homesteaded by anyone in their right mind a century ago.

So my guess is you probably don't have good soil. What is in your yard probably has too much sand, clay, limestone, or the like. This is also why I recommended that you keep your growing soil confined to raised beds—so it's separate from the poor-quality soil that probably came with your home. You'll have a well-defined boundary between good and poor soil rather than a hazy boundary of marginally good soil.

Feeding Your Soil

One time I was on a radio show and a young couple called in with a question. They had started a garden and were delighted by how much it produced for the first year or two. But after a while the plants didn't produce anything anymore. Could I tell them what was wrong? My first question to them was "What are you feeding your soil?" They were shocked by my question. You have to feed the soil? You can't just keep replanting and taking more and more food out of the garden forever and never give anything back? They didn't understand the concept of natural nutrient cycles.

Even if you are one of the lucky ones and have good soil in your backyard, you still need to keep working with it to keep it productive. The same thing is true for the soil in raised beds, even though you've started with something very high quality.

So how do you get that kind of high-nutrient soil? And how do you maintain it? The answers are simple and surprisingly easy. (And you don't need Brandon's horses.)

Let's get started.

The Basic Recipe for Compost

There are many, many ways to grow great soil. And a beautiful fact is that humans, working with nature, can create soils about 7 to 10 times faster than nature does it on her own.

Oh, I wish this book could be long enough to go over all the many different ways you can make soil and create fertility! But for the purposes of this book, I'll just go over a basic beginner system that can be done in any climate by anyone with a backyard.

The key to great soil is primarily compost. Compost fixes almost everything. Compost adds much-needed nutrients and life to every soil. It does so much more, too. Got a heavy clay soil? Compost will help open it, allowing for air and roots to move through. Got sandy soil? Compost will help hold moisture and cohesiveness. Got a rocky soil? Compost adds more organic matter and space for plant roots.

Everyone should have a compost system. There's no magic to it—besides the kind of magic you encounter on a walk through the woods as leaves, branches, and other elements around you naturally break down and decay—and there's not a lot of work you have to put into it. Yes, you're going to participate in the process, but it is a natural thing that wants to happen anyway, so nature does most of the work. Because they're the result of a natural process, compost piles are really easy ways to improve your soil—and I mean *really easy.*

I'll help you speed the process along, but even if you do everything "wrong," you really can't kill a compost pile. The worst you can do is slow it down.

Ingredients

An area for the system with a bin or composting structure

Browns—high-carbon sources (see page 100)

Greens—high-nitrogen sources (see page 100)

Air

Water

Microbes

Making Good Compost

Making compost is super simple. In your designated area, start collecting and combining your ingredients, mixing the browns with the greens, adding some microbes, and keeping the pile moist. Be sure there is always a good lining of browns at the bottom of the pile and a covering of browns on the top. Toss in new browns and greens, layer them on a regular basis, and always ensure you have a covering of browns on the top.

Keep adding materials until the pile gets fairly big and then let it sit and finish. At this point, you can start a new, separate pile. About the time you're finished building the second pile, the first will likely be ready to use. Spread the finished compost around your garden or other plants, and wait for the magic to happen. While you wait, go back to the pile you just pulled from and repeat the process, again and again, rotating between the two piles.

How long does it take to make compost? The answer is highly variable and depends on the size of your compost pile, what's in it, the size of the pieces, the moisture level, the ambient temperature, and so on. Composting can take anywhere from a couple of weeks to a couple of years. Typically, it's about a year for most piles.

Because we're aiming for the shorter end of that estimate, here are some tips to hurry things up:

- Use small pieces so they break down faster.

- Create a large pile so it will heat up more.

- Use a good mix of materials (greens and browns).

- Turn the pile to speed things up.

- Keep the pile moist; don't let it dry out or get waterlogged.

- Avoid wood chips and harder, chunkier things.

- Compost in warm weather.

How do you know when it's done? The compost should have cooled down and be dark brown and crumbly. It will smell rich, like good earth. If there are some bigger chunks that haven't finished yet, you can sift them out and put them in the second pile to finish. Or simply toss them into the garden as a part of the top dressing like I do. One exception to this is if I'm making a soil blend for seed starting. In that case, I want the compost to be fine and light, and I'll remove anything chunky.

Where should you put your compost pile? You probably don't want your compost pile in full view of the neighbors. But you also don't want to walk a half an acre to get to it. It needs to be near a source of water. A shaded area is generally better. But in the end, a compost pile works best wherever you'll actually use it. And that usually is right next to the garden.

The Three-Bay Composting System

I like my composting system to have three bays. One is for the active compost pile, one is for the finishing pile, and the third is for a stockpile of browns.

The things you add to the active pile on a day-to-day basis tend to be the greens. The third bay is there because it is very handy to have a large pile of browns on hand to add in easily and quickly. If you are going to make an error, it is much better to err on the side of having too many browns in your pile rather than too many greens.

Your compost pile should only smell like dried leaves or fresh dirt. If it's got a strange odor or it's attracting pests, mix in a lot more browns to clear up the problem very quickly. On the other hand, if nothing seems to be happening with your pile and you have gone overboard with the browns, add some greens and watch it speed up. Just play with it. You really can't hurt anything.

Each of the three bays should be approximately 4 feet by 4 feet. You can make it smaller if your yard is small, but this size is manageable for most people and lets you build up enough composting mass to really generate heat. Many people like to use wood pallets for the walls of their compost bays, and that 4-feet by 4-feet dimension just so happens to match the size of most pallets. The pallets define the borders, keep the compost out of sight, allow for airflow, and give you easy access to the material inside. You can often pick wooden pallets up for free at your local hardware or furniture store, or from a school's maintenance department. Be aware that some pallets are treated with chemicals to make them last longer. These pallets will eventually break down, releasing those chemicals into your compost. Pallets stamped HT (heat treated) or KD (kiln dried) are safe to use.

If using pallets isn't appealing, you can make your composting areas more aesthetically attractive by using wooden latticework panels or other decorative wall structures. Just be sure the walls are not solid.

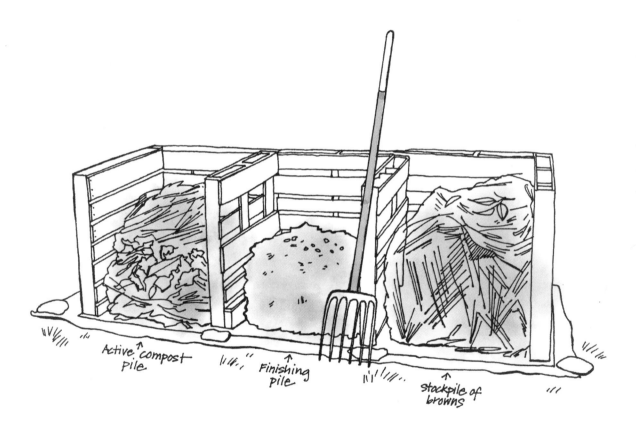

Just as you did when building your raised beds, remove all the grass and weeds from the area under and around where you want your compost to be, and line the bottom of the bays with heavy landscape cloth or several layers of cardboard. Having a good, grass-free border is important. Sometimes the heat and volume of the compost smother out the weeds, but grass is amazingly hardy and would love the challenge of growing super huge thanks to all the food in your compost pile.

I also like to put a bit of easy-to-open fencing in front of the composting bays to keep out marauding chickens and dogs. This tip comes from experience. Years ago, I had a dog named Chester who was getting fatter and fatter although I was cutting down his food to almost nothing. And I also noticed my compost pile wasn't ever getting bigger no matter how much stuff I put in it. Duh! Yes, dogs love to eat almost everything. Your compost pile will become a favorite place for them if you don't fence them out. Conversely, you don't need to fence your dogs out if you want to cut down on buying dog food.

Fancy Composting

If you are short on space and have the funds, a manufactured composter might be for you. I love to experiment with garden gadgets and have found the Aerobin 2000 composter to be a self-contained composting bin that works very well at my Colorado farmhouse. It has a unique internal core that allows airflow and speeds up composting. It fits in a small area yet is a good size for an individual or even a small family.

I have played around with compost tumblers, too, which were all the rage a while ago. The tumblers have a storage drum suspended above the ground and a handle to let you easily rotate your compost. They make turning your compost super easy, but they're also expensive and usually don't hold very much material. I haven't found the tumblers that useful. If you have physical limitations, or if someone wants to buy you one as a birthday present, go for it! Otherwise, I think you'll get more out of a more traditional setup.

The Easiest Composting System Ever

If bins sound like too much work, or if you want to follow nature's approach, just pick a spot and pile your compost on the ground. Seriously! The walls are mostly for our benefit anyway. Nature doesn't care. Walls do help hold in a little more heat, speeding up the decomposition process in colder months, but they're largely aesthetic.

Turning your compost isn't strictly necessary, but it helps speed up the process. Using a shovel, manually move all the materials around. This aerates the compost and encourages more mixing of browns and greens. Ideally, you should do this once a week, and water the pile while you're at it, to keep those microbes healthy and happy.

Does that sound like too much work? Then skip it. In reality, I almost never turn my compost piles. Like I said, your compost will break down no matter what you do. You won't stop it by neglecting to turn it over.

It really is that simple. Compost is ready whenever it feels, looks, and smells like dark, rich earth, rather than rotting scraps of food, plants, and paper. Mix it right in with your garden soil—the more, the better.

indoor composting

What if your outdoor space is limited? Bring your compost bin indoors! I know it sounds a little wild, but you can create an indoor worm farm easily and in a small space. Worm castings are the best fertilizer. Even if you have a larger outdoor composting system, you might want an indoor worm farm just for the amazing fertilizer.

Having a worm farm indoors makes a lot of sense because worms tend to like the same temperatures you and I do and aren't as happy outdoors with larger temperature swings. Several home worm farms are commercially available, or you can easily make your own. Store a bin under your sink or in a closet, introduce some worms, and add materials like you would to an outdoor bin. Worms are a little bit fussier—they don't like citrus, bread, or anything oily, for example—but otherwise, treat it like you would an outdoor bin.

I had a small worm farm at the school where I volunteered, and the kids loved it. It inspired one of the other parents to start a small business raising worms and selling worm castings.

Browns and Greens

When people talk about composting, they usually talk about the ideal ratio of browns to greens. The truth is that everything you put in your compost pile will have some carbon and some nitrogen, and determining the exact ratios in your compost pile is probably impossible and, thankfully, unnecessary.

Browns—Carbon Sources

This is the easy part. "Browns" are dried, crispy materials that are higher in carbon. Here are the classics:

- Leaves
- Old hay
- Dried grass clippings
- Shredded cardboard
- Used napkins and paper plates from your last family BBQ
- Old cotton, wool, or linen clothes
- Coffee filters
- Shredded paper (I have a paper shredder in my home office that creates nice browns.)
- Cardboard toilet paper and paper towel rolls
- Wood chips
- Dried, chopped tree trimmings
- Corn husks and cobs
- Pine needles
- Cardboard egg cartons torn into bits
- Old dried herbs
- Nutshells

Greens—Nitrogen Sources

The greens for your compost system start in your kitchen where you collect food scraps. I have a small decorative bucket (with a lid) on my countertop. Some people have containers under their cabinets, but I prefer a smaller bucket on the counter-top because it is more convenient. Emptying the compost bucket is a daily, or every other day, chance to get outside and visit your chickens and garden. Having it on the counter just makes it easy to grab and go.

Honestly, a lot of kitchen scraps won't make it to the compost system because your chickens will love to eat them. And if you have dogs, they will like to eat the miscellaneous meat bits the chickens wouldn't really like. But there are times when you will have scraps neither wants, such as coffee grounds or fruit rinds, and these are great to toss on the compost pile. Here is a list of other possible greens:

- Used coffee grounds
- Fresh-cut grass clippings
- Green garden weeds
- Old and outdated foods (from the freezer or pantry)
- Hair and nail clippings
- Fruit rinds
- Eggshells
- Chicken manure (from the coop)
- Rabbit pellets
- Spent bouquets of flowers

- Stale bread
- Old pasta or rice
- Seaweed
- Rotted fruits or vegetables (I have a lot of these at my Puerto Rico property.)
- Meats and grease (See note.)
- Fish carcasses (See note.)
- Dairy products (See note.)
- Urine (See note.)

note: Meats, grease, fish carcasses, and dairy products are often not recommended for compost piles, and you may want to skip them as a beginner. Most of the time my dogs prefer to eat these items, so they rarely have a chance to make it to the compost pile. But still, I am in the category of growers who compost pretty much everything. My philosophy is just mix it up with enough browns, water it in, and it will be fine. Also—and this one may freak out some of you—your urine is an excellent source of nitrogen and a whole lot of other minerals you excrete. If you want to use it to soak your compost pile, I recommend you dilute it to 1 part urine to 10 parts water.

Other materials, like wax, bones, larger branches, and cedarwood take longer to break down, but you can still add them to your compost pile. You may need to sort them out and leave them behind when you distribute the rest of your finished compost.

Here are items that should *not* go into the compost pile:

- Styrofoam
- Plastic wrap
- Tape on boxes or cardboard
- Household cleaners
- Sawdust from treated wood
- Ash from burned coal
- Sticky labels from fruits or vegetables
- Heavily coated or colored magazine or packaging
- Cat and dog feces
- Diseased plants

A small amount of ash from your fireplace or wood-burning stove is okay—of course, be sure there are no ashes still lit—but you don't want to go overboard with it.

Air

Your compost pile needs air. One of the reasons you want to have a lot of browns is that they are usually light and fluffy and allow space for air to circulate. The need for air is also the reason the sides of your compost bays should not be solid, but rather pallets, wire mesh, or wood lattice. If you decide to regularly turn your compost, you are essentially adding more air, or oxygen, to the bacteria that are doing the work, and oxygen is fuel for them. This is why turning the pile accelerates the composting process.

Water

The compost pile needs to stay moist but not soggy. The bacteria doing the work cannot live in a very dry environment. The pile will need to be watered regularly, which is another great reason why it should be near your garden. You are already watering your garden anyway, so it's a simple thing to turn the watering wand and give the compost pile a spritz.

The water you use is also important. As discussed in earlier chapters, municipal water usually has heavy chemicals like chlorine and chloramine to kill bacteria. This is directly going against what you are trying to achieve in your compost pile. It's the bacteria and microorganisms that do the composting, and you don't want to kill those guys! Collected rainwater, water pumped from a small pond, or well water are better choices in general. If all you have is municipal water, I recommend you use a filtering system that will remove as much of the bacteria-killing chlorine and chloramine as possible.

Microbes

The cutting edge for agriculture in the twenty-first century is soil microbiology. There is just so much we don't know—but what we do know is pretty exciting. I've talked a bit already about the beneficial relationships between plants and the life in the soil, and there is so much more amazing research going on right now. For example, groups are working to figure out how to remediate overly chemically toxic soils using special strains of fungi and other microbiology. As a beginner, you'll get to join in the fun by encouraging more microbial life in your compost piles, garden soils, and more.

So how do you get those microbes working for you in your compost? Actually, if you do absolutely nothing at all, there are already plenty of microbes in the compost, and the pile will eventually take off on its own. But it does help if you inoculate the pile. That is pretty simple to do. Take at least a couple of handfuls—several shovelfuls is better—of rich, active soil from somewhere else, and mix it into your compost pile. Simply sprinkle the soil in between the layers of browns and greens, and water it well. You can get that starter soil from a friend who has a pile or dig a bit from a forest or greenbelt. Or you may find a small area in your own yard where leaves have been accumulating, and underneath that will be a nice, vibrant little patch of soil that is brimming with life. Those microbes would love to be in your compost pile.

You can also pick up a bottle of soil microbe inoculant at your local garden store. Some people brew a special "compost tea," which is basically a brew rich with nutrients and microbes that are great for inoculating compost piles and to add directly to the garden soil. Ask around at a local garden club, and I'm sure you'll find a compost tea enthusiast who will share some with you.

when do you use the compost?

How often do you apply the finished compost to your garden? A rough guideline is to add a good 2 inches of compost to the garden bed at the beginning of every growing season just before you plant. During each growing season, scatter a handful or two of compost around the plants' roots for an extra boost.

the soil-gut connection

What do your garden and your gut have in common? Microbes! A teaspoon of rich garden soil can contain a billion microbes. A healthy human intestinal tract can contain 100 trillion bacterial cells, or around 277 billion per inch.

Probiotic bacteria are essential for our health, and they find their way into our gut through our foods. But without good soil, the whole system breaks down.

Soils in America are disappearing at a rate 10 times faster than they are naturally replenished. By growing your own food, you can help reverse this trend. Not only are you preserving soil, you're also helping replenish it hundreds of times faster than if nature was acting alone.

Buying vs. Creating Compost

You might be wondering if you can buy compost instead of creating it. Yes, you can . . . but I don't think you'll want to. Earlier, I encouraged you to buy good soil because it lets you start right away, so you can avoid the time it takes to build it up. It's a one-time purchase and the fastest path to success. But compost will be a regular addition to your garden, and there are several good reasons to make your own:

- Creating your own compost gives you more independence. You don't have to depend on your local garden store staying in business or worry about contamination from external inputs.

- Buying compost costs money. Making compost is free.

- Making compost is easy. At the bare minimum, it's piling organic materials on the ground and walking away. Even if you do nothing, and give no attention to the brown-to-green ratio, it will still break down.

- Making compost is environmentally friendly. You're going to have yard waste anyway. Rather than bagging it up and leaving it out for the trash collectors, why not let it break down in your own yard and return those nutrients to the soil?

But the best reason of all to DIY instead of buy is that your own homemade compost can be infinitely better than store-bought. It goes back to the soil microbiology. Most commercial compost is made from a limited number of inputs. Your compost is going to have many, many different types of ingredients—all that different vegetable waste, hair, coffee grinds, and so on. The more diverse the ingredient sources, the more diverse the population of soil microbes that can be supported, and the greater likelihood of a wider variety of available nutrients. Also, your own homemade compost is fresh and bursting with life, instead of sitting in plastic bags on a dock or in a warehouse for weeks.

It All Starts with the Soil

When I visited with the Tarahumara Indians of Mexico's Copper Canyon, I brought many gifts. One was a bag of commercially grown corn. The Tarahumara politely refused the corn and explained that my corn would not give them the strength their own homegrown corn gave them. They showed me their fields where they grew their corn and explained their very simple yet effective system for creating their unique soil. The children tended a herd of goats that were pastured in the surrounding mountains during the day and penned up at night. The goat droppings in the pen were composted, and that compost was applied to the soil each year before the corn was planted. Additionally, during the growing season, a handful of the compost was added to each plant. The fields we were standing in had been producing corn with this system for hundreds of years.

We are quickly losing the traditional practices of the Tarahumara and other land-tenders, and as a result, we are also nearing "peak soil," the alarmingly fast rate at which we're losing the fertile soil necessary to sustain the world's populations. There are many reasons for this, but the biggest culprits are industrial food production and conventional agricultural practices. According to the World Wildlife Fund, about half of the world's topsoil has been lost in the last 150 years. There is a deep concern for humanity's ability to feed itself in the very near future.

Don't underestimate the value you contribute when you grow your own food and create your own compost. Producing your own food takes some pressure off the commercial systems, and making your compost creates soil fertility. What you do is important and necessary.

Once you get going, your whole backyard can become a healthy ecosystem in its own right, with all the different parts and pieces supporting one another. All this leads to less waste, more nutritious food, a stronger environment overall, and a healthier and hardier you, which is a pretty amazing outcome you make with your own hands! Your health is your greatest asset and much more valuable than anything else you can own or buy. Creating compost is a system for true wealth, and it all starts with the soil.

chapter summary

- Great soil, teeming with life, is the secret to a green thumb.

- Your nutrition ultimately comes from the soil your food is grown in.

- Health is your greatest asset.

- Your own homemade compost will be much richer in nutrients, life, and vitality than any commercially produced compost.

- You can compost almost anything if it once was alive.

- You and I are a part of a never-ending cycle of life that involves a complex web of mutually beneficial giving and receiving.

- You can't mess up compost. You can only slow it down.

- Growing your own food and building soil is an important contribution to your children and the entire planet.

additional resources

For more information on nurturing soil, check out these websites:

- www.FreeFertilizers.com. A free ebook with 50 homemade fertilizers.

- www.FunnyCompostMovie.com. A movie created by David the Good that will have you laughing all the way to new methods of creating compost. Spoiler: The best line from the movie is about how to compost your enemies.

- www.TarahumaraCorn.com. Two in-depth videos filmed during my time with the Tarahumara Indians. Learn how to grow, process, and cook their corn. You'll get to see the fields and the goats, and meet the farmer and his kids. Beautiful videography and stunning images.

- www.CompostingColors.com. Can you compost colored magazines and newspapers? A very lively and interesting discussion on this topic is going on here, with the latest information on the toxicity (or not) of various inks, materials, and printing processes.

chapter 6

foraging and
wild tending

The modern concept of "wilderness" is tragically flawed. When John Muir, an influential environmentalist and founder of the Sierra Club, looked over the beautiful beds of gold and purple flowers in the Central Valley of California, he thought he was looking at pristine, untouched wilderness. Certainly, there were no people anywhere, and he believed this abundance of food and stunning beauty must be what the land reverted to when left untouched by humans. But nothing could be further from the truth. Other Europeans before him had brought diseases that decimated the population of indigenous peoples in advance of Muir's arrival.

Prior to the arrival of the Europeans, the native Miwok and Yokut Indians had been carefully tending the land for millennia with controlled burns, planting, harvesting, and seeding. Many modern people assume hunter-gatherers just walked around randomly and ate whatever they could find, but earlier peoples had an intimate relationship with and knew minute details about every aspect of their territories.

I was on a desert wilderness trip with David Holliday, an expert in Stone Age living skills, when the subject of how to find water came up. We were learning how to recognize the plants and other landscape clues that indicated springs or streams were nearby. David told me that children in earlier ages would not have been taught how to identify where water was. "Why not?" I asked. "That seems like an essential skill." David laughed and said, "If you wanted to know where water was, all you had to do was ask your grandmother."

Much of this knowledge has been lost over time, but nature continues to be a truly miraculous dance that propagates all kinds of life. Here's just one example: most seeds of fruit-bearing plants are designed with just enough protection to go through the digestive tract of animals. The animal eats the seeds, carries them away, and deposits them in a nice package of fertilizer (poop) in other locations. I'm sure you've noticed fence lines where birds have planted trees and bushes from the berries they've eaten and deposited. These kinds of interactions are everywhere. Many people know about the example of bees who go after nectar and inadvertently fertilize flowers with the pollen on their legs. There are literally millions upon millions of these relationships and dependencies in the complex web of life.

Likewise, an appropriate number of humans harvesting and tending is very beneficial to the health of the land. I had the opportunity to see this up close when I spent some time with Nikki Hill, a modern-day wild tender. Nikki showed me how to harvest the breadroot plant that grows on the high desert mesas (*Lonatium* and *Cymopterus* genus). The best time to harvest the yummy root is when the seeds are ripe. As Nikki explained, when you dig and disturb the hard-packed ground to get at the roots, the seeds fall from the plant into the soil you just loosened. So as you are harvesting, you are also planting. Without humans working the soil, the seeds still fall, but they often aren't viable on the hard ground. The plants need to be harvested to survive. Nikki showed me some small patches of breadroot that are remnants of what used to be vast areas of wild-cultivated food.

Humans working consciously can dramatically increase soil, biodiversity, and overall productivity more than nature can do on her own. We are a surprisingly important part of the natural process.

the truth about "living off the land"

Some people have an almost romantic dream of returning to a pure hunter-gatherer lifestyle. I often hear this from people concerned about a collapse of civilization. The idea is that no matter what happens, you can always take your rifle and a few supplies and head out to the wilderness to live off the land. But at the end of the day, this is a completely unrealistic, untenable way of life for many us. We need community and companionship to survive and thrive.

If you were to pack up and leave, though, you would need to know how much land it takes to support a person without destroying all the wildlife and plant populations. How much area do you need to live sustainably as a hunter-gatherer?

Because there are so few actual hunter-gatherers left on the planet, and the few places where they do still exist tend to be jungles that look nothing like North America, let's turn to anthropological data. The quick and easy answer is that traditional peoples used, on average, about 10 square miles of resources per person to survive; 10 square miles is 6,400 acres— just for one person. Numerous studies validate this number. One of the most accessible books that describes this in more detail is Jared Diamond's book *Collapse: How Societies Choose to Fail or Succeed.*

Of course, this average living land varied by area of the country. California's lush and diverse landscapes were able to support some of the highest native-population densities known in North America—1.5 people per square mile lived on the coast of the Santa Barbara channel. At the other end of the spectrum, the desert regions of California held roughly 1 person per 12.5 square miles. There's some debate about these numbers because this study raises a lot of questions about how many people Earth can really support. But it does show that, should we all decide to be hunter-gatherers in today's world, our planet could not withstand it.

The great news is that you don't need to become a hunter-gatherer to be self-sufficient. As I've shown you in the preceding chapters, you can grow at least half of your own food in a backyard-sized space—and do it in a way that is beneficial to you and to the land. And you know what? You can probably grow a lot more. The Grow System assumes you are a beginner. As your skills and system expand, you'll be able to produce even more in smaller and smaller areas. So focus on your primary source of food from the intensive systems you implement in your backyard, and incorporate some wild tending and foraging as a complement.

The Importance of Food Variety

Why is eating some wild foods important for you?

Eating a wide variety of foods, including wild foods, ensures that you get all the macro- and micronutrients you need. Around the world, indigenous diets were incredibly diverse, consisting of thousands of different species each year. Contrast that with the contemporary American diet. How many species of animals and plants does the typical grocery store shopper eat? For plants, we can count the big five: rice, wheat, corn, soy, and potatoes. Toss in a fast-food hamburger, and we can add tomatoes, onions, pickles (cucumber), and iceberg lettuce (an utterly empty food, but we'll still count it). The rest will vary, but most Americans eat only around 12 vegetables. For meats, most people eat exclusively beef, pork, and chicken. We might find a couple of species of fish as well—perhaps catfish, salmon, or tilapia. Dairy products come from cows, which is a species we've already mentioned, and eggs come from chickens. We know most livestock are primarily fed corn, wheat, soy, and other unmentionables derived from corn, wheat, or soy. So that brings the total species that most Americans consume on a regular basis to around 12.

Let's talk about corn a little more. Corn is the biggest crop the United States produces, and it is a huge part of our diet. Chemical food engineers, who specialize in creating the ingredients and flavors for processed food, have figured out so many creative ways to slice and dice corn molecules and include them in all kinds of products. Todd Dawson, a plant biologist at the University of California-Berkeley, can determine how much corn is in a person's diet by analyzing hair samples for a particular form of carbon found in corn. Dawson's testing has revealed that the carbon in an average American body is 70 percent corn. "We are like corn chips with legs," says Dawson.

Oh, how could I have forgotten chocolate and coffee? Okay, let's call it 14 species.

Is it any wonder that so many of us are chronically sick? Humans are omnivores. We are the ultimate generalists. How can we expect to be healthy by eating only 14 different foods?

A diversity of foods supports a diversity of gut microbes. And those gut microbes are a huge part of our immune systems. They also produce neurotransmitters that are essential to our mental health. Can you imagine how robust and diverse your gut flora would be if you ate 1,000 different species each year? It's similar to why your homemade compost is so much better than store-bought compost. As discussed in Chapter 5, homemade compost is superior because of its diversity of ingredients, which provide for the growth of a huge diversity of microbes. Never underestimate the raw power of microbial diversity!

Most people don't realize just how powerful wild foods are. The plants and animals we buy at the grocery store have been bred for aesthetics. They are grown so that they are bigger, look nicer on a shelf, and have an increased shelf life. The foods you create in your home systems will have a huge increase in quality and diversity. But undomesticated foods take this to the next level. They have additional potencies that can radically benefit your health.

Nature does not select for aesthetics (except where reproduction is involved). Nature selects for survival. Wild plants and animals have passed through countless generations of development and refinement to bring them to the pinnacle of efficiency and nutrient density. They aren't being tended by a kindly gardener or farmer. No one is supplementing their feed with extra minerals or ensuring they are well watered and in an ideal environment. Wild animals and plants have to work for a living, and they have to be good at it. This makes them incredibly adaptable and strong, and when you eat them, they pass that strength to you.

Identifying Plants

You know the best place to learn about wild plants? Your own backyard. Seriously, those "weeds," like dandelion, thistle, or mallow, have a lot to offer you. If you don't know what those plants look like, don't worry. The first step in becoming a forager and wild tender is learning a bit about botany. You need to know some basic plant biology to positively identify plants, differentiate them from poisonous lookalikes, and learn common uses of larger groups of plants. In this chapter, we look at a few of the identifying characteristics and some of the common, easily identifiable families.

These days, numerous apps can help you identify plants right on your phone. Although the apps are getting better at recognizing and identifying plants, I wouldn't want to trust my life to them. Beyond that, learning to identify plants deepens your understanding and appreciation of them. By studying the terms and their meanings, you empower yourself to understand plants in new and deeper ways. They become a part of you, and a dead battery or "no service" area can never take that away. It's like the difference between being fluent in a language and using a translator.

Although it often looks haphazard and random, every plant has a particular pattern for how it would like to grow. The plant often doesn't get to achieve its ideal form due to blocked sunlight, grazing animals, or a zillion other factors. But there is a clear, underlying pattern. How the leaves grow, the shape of the flowers, the root structure, and every other aspect of a plant has a built-in way of manifesting, and this is what you can learn to recognize. A good reference is the book *Botany in a Day: The Patterns Method of Plant Identification* by Thomas Elpel. I will forewarn you that Elpel's title is somewhat misleading—it takes a bit more than a day to really learn botany—but he has done a great job to help simplify the process.

Leaves: Alternate and Opposite

Let's start by looking at leaves. Two of the most common leaf patterns you will encounter are alternate and opposite. An alternate leaves arrangement is the most common, and you'll find it on many plants. The leaves grow in a back-and-forth pattern. One leaf grows out of the stem on one side, then, a little farther down the stem, another leaf grows out of the other side. They do not come out together at the same point on the stem. Garden plants with alternate leaves include sweet potatoes, okra, pumpkins, and squash.

Opposite leaves are less common. They come together at the same point on a stem, but they come out on opposite sides, as the name implies. Your herb garden is a great place to find examples. Lavender, peppermint, and oregano all have opposite leaves.

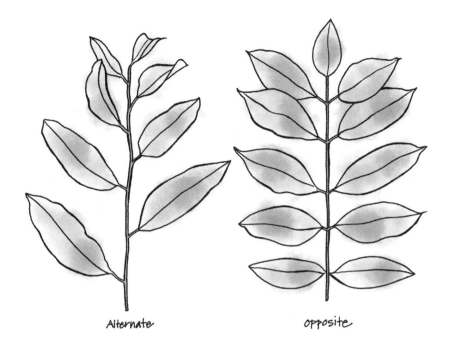

Alternate   opposite

Venation: Net and Parallel

Next, let's talk about veins. Go out and look at the veins on the leaves of plants around you. Leaf veins come in many variations, but the two basic categories are net and parallel. The most common is net venation, where the veins have an intersecting pattern that resembles a net. Tomato, squash, pumpkins, melons, and okra all have a net venation pattern.

Parallel leaf veins do not branch. They run parallel to one another, without criss-crossing. Corn, onions, garlic, grasses, plantains, and leeks all have a parallel venation.

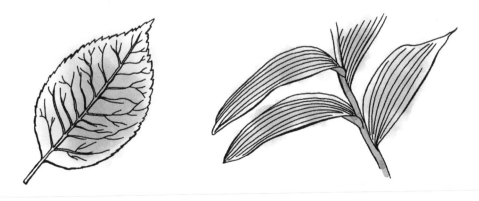

When you go out and start looking at the plants in your yard and garden, you will come across lots of other formations. Don't worry about them for now, but do begin to notice them. Try to find some alternate and opposite leaf attachments and then try to find some net and parallel venation. These are the most common, and I'm sure you'll find some plants with these in your yard. When you think you've found them, congratulate yourself and know you've got a high five from me. You have a lot more to learn for sure, but you've taken your first step.

Life Cycles: Annuals, Biannuals, and Perennials

Sometimes plants are grouped by their life cycles, which come in three rough categories:

Annuals. Annuals are plants that grow, make seeds, and die all within a single year, or even a single season. Almost all your garden vegetables are annuals. Cucumbers, squash, watermelon, zucchini, pumpkins, and most species of sunflowers are annuals.

Biannuals. Biannuals are plants that live for 2 years. This is easy to remember because "bi" means "two" and "annual" refers to a year. The name literally means "2 years." Carrots, garlic, parsley, and kale are all biannual plants.

Perennials. Perennials live 3 or more years. Blueberries, strawberries, and nut and fruit trees are all perennials. Potatoes are perennials, too, although you might not guess it at first. The foliage dies back, but the tuber waits patiently in the ground, ready to produce new leaves when conditions are right. You interrupt the plant's plans by digging up and eating the tubers.

Some plants are grown as annuals in colder areas, but they can live as perennials in tropical areas. Tomatoes, okra, and peppers can all live as perennials if they are protected from cold weather.

Flowers and Plant Families

Plants are grouped into families, and often (but not always) members of the family tend to have similar medicinal and edible characteristics. Which family a plant belongs in is determined by its flower. Why the flower and not the leaves, or roots, or stem? Because the flowers are the sex parts of the plant. An organism's sex parts determine who it can share genetic material with, and they can also be used to determine the organism's phylogenetic family. For example, rabbits are rabbits because they cannot mate with cats or dogs.

Following is a diagram of the parts of a flower. It's good general knowledge to know the names of the parts, but sometimes it can be tricky to identify them in nature. So many natural variations of flowers exist, and humans have bred many different kinds of flowers, too. It can be a little frustrating, but it does get easier as you go along.

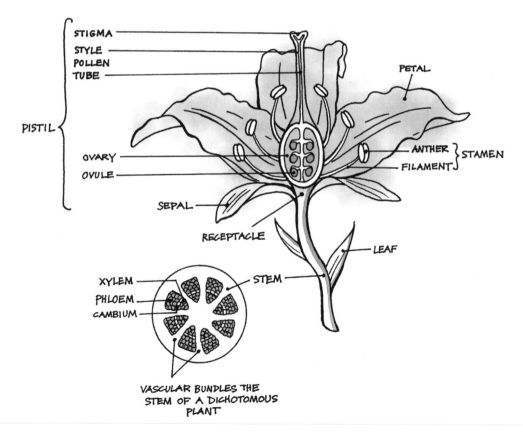

The absolute best way to learn about plants is to get familiar with what you are growing in your garden. You already know what your plants are, so the identification part is done for you. Let's take a look at six plant families you may see growing in the wild and be able to use for foraging.

Brassicaceae

The mustard family. Broccoli, brussels sprouts, cauliflower, kale, and cabbage are all members of this family. The leaves and flowers of these are all edible in some way, although they often have a powerful flavor.

Mustard flowers always have four petals. Hiding behind the petals are four sepals. These leaflike structures are usually green but may be other colors. At the center of the flower are six stamens (the male part of the flower) around one pistil (the female part of the flower). Four of the stamens are tall, and two are short.

The flowers are usually small, and you may need a magnifying lens to see the details. They are arranged in a spiraling cluster called a raceme.

Solanaceae

The nightshade family. This family includes both edible and toxic members. If you grow tomatoes, potatoes, peppers, or eggplant, you're growing a member of the nightshade family. Nightshade blooms have parts in fives: five united petals, five united sepals, and five stamens. Tomatoes sometimes buck this trend, due to hybridization.

Fabaceae

The pea family. In this family, its flower is the key to identification. Pea flowers have a very distinctive bloom pattern called the "banner, wings, and keel."

Across the top of the bloom is the banner. This is a single petal that stretches across the bloom like the sail of a ship or . . . well, a banner. At both sides are the wings. These are each a single petal that may stretch out to the side or curve around to follow the "keel." The keel is the bottom of the bloom, and it's made up of two petals that are usually fused into one. They stick out like the keel of a ship. Together, the bloom may remind you of a little boat with a sail and two paddles at the side. To see this in your garden, take a look at any of your peas or beans.

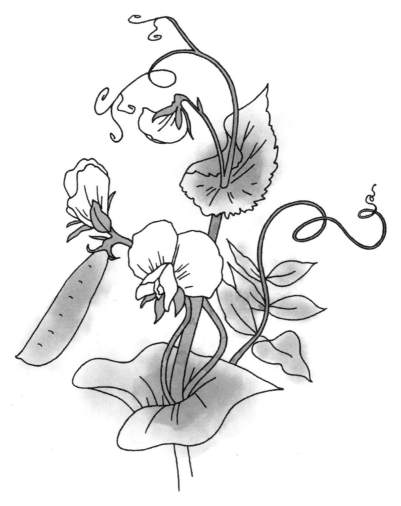

Most members of this family are safe, especially when cooked. There are a few that are mildly poisonous, such as locoweed and lupine, and very few that are significantly dangerous, such as wisteria and the rosary pea.

Lamiaceae

The mint family. The mint family is most easily recognized by its square stems, opposite leaves, and aromatic smell. The pairs of opposite leaves also rotate around the stem. For example, if one pair of leaves came out to the east and west, the next pair would come out to the north and south.

Mint blooms have five petals, but the top four are fused together. Only the bottom petal is separate. The overall appearance is like a tube with lips at the end. Mint flowers have four stamens.

As long as a plant follows the pattern of the mint family *and* has an aromatic smell, it's not toxic.

Many of our culinary herbs and herbal teas come from the mint family. Naturally, peppermint and spearmint are mints. You'll also find oregano, lavender, rosemary, lemon balm, thyme, savory, patchouli, and basil in this family. And if you've ever grown a chia pet, you were actually growing a member of the mint family.

Rosaceae

The rose family. Rose family flowers have five petals with five sepals and numerous stamens. They are often very aromatic. The rose family gives us quite a lot of food, too. Apples, peaches, pears, plums, cherries, strawberries, blackberries, raspberries, almonds, apricots, and nectarines are all in the rose family. Oh, and roses, too!

Poaceae

The grass family. Grasses are usually wind pollinated. Their flowers are small and do not have showy petals, but they still have stamens and pistils like other flowers. These plants all have parallel leaf veins and form a seed stalk that's hollow in the middle, except at the nodes.

Most grasses are safe to eat, although a few can be problematic. The biggest danger with the grasses isn't the plant itself, but a fungus called ergot. Ergot can cause hallucinations and other health problems in humans. Avoid plants with discolored grains.

All our grains are grasses, including wheat, rice, barley, rye, oats, and millet. But the most common grass to have in your garden is corn. Yes, corn is just big grass that has dedicated so much of itself to partnership with humanity that it grows a huge seed head and sacrifices almost everything else.

Growing Location

In addition to all the various parts of the plants, the location where it is growing is often a way to identify it. For example, the breadroot plant Nikki taught me to harvest is in the Apiaceae family. This family includes a lot of wonderful edibles, such as carrots, parsley, cilantro, and celery. But when I grow those plants, I always grow from a known seed source. I never forage for any species in the Apiaceae family because it also contains the poisonous hemlock plant. Hemlock, you might recall, was in the drink they made Socrates take for the death penalty. I know I don't have the knowledge to identify the difference between a wild carrot and poison hemlock, so I avoid that family completely. But Nikki showed me that hemlock only grows close to water such as streams or rivers. And the breadroot only grows in very dry areas. So the location of where the plant is growing is also a huge part of identifying it.

harvesting safely

When you are looking for wild edibles, it's very important that you proceed cautiously. Here are some guidelines:

- Always consult three different sources to confirm a plant's identity and edibility.

- Gather plants only during the daytime. Poor lighting greatly increases the chances that you'll misidentify a plant and harvest the wrong thing.

- Start small. When you try a new plant for the first time, always start with a tiny portion. Even if the plant is edible, you may have a sensitivity or allergy to it.

- For maximum safety, use the Universal Edibility Test. At the end of the chapter, I include a link to a free ebook that will walk you through the test step-by-step.

harvesting respectfully

My friend Nicole Telkes used to work for the American Botanical Council (ABC), a fine organization dedicated to the responsible use of medicinal plants. Nicole's job was to write a monthly monograph about a specific herb. But both Nicole and ABC ended the project when they realized that after a monograph was published on a wild herb, it would be the kiss of death for that herb because so many people would go out and overharvest it.

Harvesting but not overharvesting is a delicate balance, and you have to know how much of any plant to take without causing problems. Some plants are weedy, so you can take a lot and not bother the resiliency of the stand; some plants, such as the breadroot, love the interaction and thrive with human harvesting; others can be overharvested easily. I strongly recommend you focus on the abundant weedy species for your first harvests. And in general, when you are gathering wild edibles, remember to be gentle with the land and only take what you need.

Your First Forage: Hunting for Acorns

The first foraging plant I want to introduce you to is super safe and one I am sure you are already familiar with—the oak tree. Oak trees come in different sizes and different shapes, and they have different-looking leaves. They do, however, all share some characteristics that can be used to identify them. Oak trees have alternate leaves with a net venation, and they are all perennial. They also have one other important characteristic in common—acorns.

I look forward to each autumn when the time is right for harvesting acorns, one of my favorite foods. One time I was traveling for business, and on my morning run, I found this awesome oak tree that was dropping acorns like crazy. The great thing was they were falling on a slightly slanted driveway, so the acorns were all rolling down and gathering together in a single spot at the edge of the street—a dream setup for harvesting. Just as I came upon this scene, the owner of the home came outside, so I politely asked her if I could collect the acorns. She narrowed her eyes at me and took an uncomfortable length of time to respond, which made me nervous. Then she said, "You *want* these annoying things?" I almost burst with joy.

Acorns are a lot of fun to gather. You get to enjoy being outdoors in the cool weather with all the smells of autumn. Be sure to share the experience with your family. If you have children, you can have acorn-throwing fights, and unlike tomato throwing, it doesn't hurt the harvest or your clothes. Making memories is a big part of the experience!

Plus, acorns are a very nutritious food, high in healthy oils and protein. Larger acorns are easier to work with, and you get more food for your effort. But all acorns are edible, so use whatever you have around you.

You need to prepare the acorns before you eat them. My favorite way to cook with them is to make an acorn meal. You can use acorn meal to cut the flour in many baking recipes. It adds a unique, nutty flavor. Or you can add it to meatloaf to stretch the hamburger. There are lots of creative ways to use acorn meal, and I would love to hear from you about your experiments with it.

To make acorn meal, follow these steps:

1. Gather the acorns that have fallen to the ground. Discard any with holes in them.

2. Float test your harvest to quickly separate the good acorns from the bad ones. Fill your sink with water, and pour in your acorns. Acorns that float are usually bad. Acorns that sink are usually good. It's as easy as that.

3. Remove the tannins by shelling. Oaks are rich in tannins, which are chemicals that have an astringent or drying effect on bodily tissues. Nearly all acorns have a tannin content that is too high for humans to eat raw.

   Start by shelling the acorns and extracting the nut meat. You can use a nut-cracker, just as you would for pecans. I usually just use a hammer.

   Discard any shriveled or moldy acorns that got past the float test. If a bad spot is small enough, you can scratch it off with a knife.

4. Make the acorn meal. Fill your blender with the acorn meat, add at least two to four times the volume of water as acorn meat, and blend it into an acorn slurry. Pour the slurry into a large canning jar, and let it sit. After an hour or two, the acorn meal will settle to the bottom and the tannin-rich water will rise to the top. Pour off the tannin water, and refill the jar with fresh water, stirring or shaking the mixture again. Repeat this 5 to 10 times or more until the tannin water gets lighter and clearer.

Another option is to pour the acorn slurry into a cloth sack or a clean sock, twist the top shut, and massage the bag under a running tap. At first, the runoff will be a cloudy brown to white. After around 15 minutes, the runoff should be a lot closer to clear. When this happens, open the bag and taste a small pinch of the acorn meal. If it is still bitter or astringent, it needs more massaging. If the bitterness is gone, squeeze out any excess water, and you've got acorn meal.

Some people also like to spread the mush across a baking sheet and put it in the oven on low heat until dry. I have no patience for drying and always want to eat the acorn meal right away, so I cook with it slightly damp. If you do dry the mush, be sure to refrigerate it after drying because acorn meal contains fatty oils that will spoil at room temperature.

Many nuts, such as pecans, can only store for about 6 months before they start going rancid, but acorns can store for many years in their shells. In their book *It Will Live Forever: Traditional Yosemite Indian Acorn Preparation*, Julia Parker and Beverly Ortiz say the best-tasting acorns are those that have been stored for 2 years. I'm still working on testing that out, and I'll keep you posted.

acorn meal "pancakes"

One of my favorite ways to eat acorn meal is to make "pancakes" out of it. I use damp acorn meal, toss in two or three eggs, a pinch of salt, and a tablespoon or two of maple syrup (optional). If I think of it, I'll add some cinnamon or allspice. I mix all that well and cook it on the stovetop in a pan with melted butter—very similar to how you cook pancakes except these are heavier, so they take a bit longer to cook. Best of all, they have so much more nutrition and flavor.

If your acorn meal still has a little bitterness, add some milk to the recipe. The milk will bind with the lingering tannins, masking their taste.

I'm a very basic cook, but for more really amazing recipes, I recommend the book *Eating Acorns* by Marcie Lee Mayer. And of course, many other acorn-related resources are on the web.

next steps

After you've mastered gathering acorns, you can move on to hunting for wild weeds. In her book *The Wild Wisdom of Weeds: 13 Essential Plants for Human Survival*, Katrina Blair features the top weeds that serve as a valuable source of food and medicine. They're all common around the world, so wherever you live, and no matter where you travel, you will always have plant friends and food.

Here are the 13 featured plants:

Amaranth (**Amaranthus spp.**).
Delicious greens and seeds.

Chickweed (**Stellaria media**).
Delicate greens with pretty star flowers.

Clover (**Trifolium pratense, T. spp.**).
Beautiful greens and blossoms.

Dandelion (**Taraxacum officinale**). The spring leaves are a satisfying bitter, and the roasted root makes a robust coffee substitute.

Dock (**Rumex crispus**). Tart and lemony.

Grass (**Poaceae family**). Whole grains for free.

Knotweed (**Polygonum aviculare**).
Spicy or mild, but always delicious.

Lambsquarter (**Chenopodium album**).
Like spinach, but better tasting and more nutritious.

Mallow (**Malva neglecta, M. spp.**). Smooth and soothing.

Mustard (**Brassicaceae family**). Hot and spicy.

Plantain (**Plantago spp.**). Bold and earthy.

Purslane (**Portulaca oleracea**).
Juicy succulent for salads or pizza topping.

Thistle (**Carduus nutans, Cirsium vulgare, Silybum marianum, Cnicus benedictus**). Green and juicy.

Incorporating Foraging and Wild Tending into Your Life

Foraging doesn't have to be limited to plants, and wild tending can take many forms. There are many creative ways to incorporate foraging and wild tending into your life.

My family goes for short vacations on the coast. Grandparents, kids, aunts, and uncles all come together for a big, fun reunion time. A few days into these trips, I go foraging down at the docks. I meet the fishing boats as they come in and hang around as the fishermen clean their fish. In the public cleaning facility, you can find all the best parts of the fish. When I pull from the discarded heads, skeletons, tails, and skins in the bin, the fishermen stare at me with those funny looks I've grown used to seeing on my in-laws' faces. But I just go on and do my work. Most of the carcasses are still cold from being in ice chests on the boats. I carefully remove the guts, cut out the gills, and thoroughly clean the remainders so I have nice, clean skeletons and heads. I take all this back to our rental and put it in a big pot with some water. I add a bunch of onions, garlic, and celery and let it simmer on the stove overnight.

The next day I pour off the deeply nutritious broth and store it in glass jars in the freezer. I use this broth to nourish my family's bodies over the coming months.

Wild tending is about using the natural resources our beautiful planet has to offer, but using them respectfully and mindfully. Tend the earth wisely.

chapter summary

- Human participation in tending the wild is a more accurate representation of what wilderness is and can be.

- Modern diets are surprisingly limited, and adding more diversity of foods you eat will increase the diversity and strength of your gut microbiome.

- Learning botany may take some time, but it gives you a superpower to find food and medicine anywhere.

- Some species of plants thrive with human interaction, and some can be destroyed. As a new forager, start with weedy, abundant species.

additional resources

For more information on foraging and wild tending, check out these websites:

- www.UniversalEdibilityTest.com. An ebook explaining the Universal Edibility Test with step-by-step instructions for determining edibility of unknown wild plants.

- www.ProcessingRoadkill.com. Another form of foraging. This free video shows you how to judge the edibility of found meat (deer, raccoon, and so on) and how to process it simply with a common knife.

- www.HandMadeShampoo.com. A free ebook that includes a list of plant species that have lots of saponins, the soapy, sudsy-like cleaning quality you can use to make your own soap from wild plants.

- www.HowToCookAcorns.com. A lively discussion at The Grow Network with lots of recipes on how to prepare acorns.

- https://TheGrowNetwork.com/academy. Online training in botany, wild tending, growing food, making medicine, and more. It includes an interactive forum with experienced homesteaders who love answering questions.

become a home
medicine-maker

chapter 7

the process:
seven stages to becoming a
medicine woman or man

ead lice. Oh, the shame. The not-so-subtle shunning by the in-laws and friends. The stigma, even though almost everyone with kids has had the same problem themselves at one time or another. Head lice is a rite of passage for many youngsters, and mine were no exception. I groaned as I learned that the recommended course of action was a foul-smelling, toxic concoction to be applied topically to my children's heads. Should I really be applying this nasty chemical to the highly absorbent scalp right near my children's brains?

Luckily, I had made the decision when my children were very young that I was going to learn about herbal medicines. I decided to become their first line of defense, rather than outsourcing that responsibility to someone else. I wasn't an expert yet, but I had learned enough that I thought I could handle this. And I knew I didn't want to apply poison to my children's heads and then isolate them from all human contact.

After doing some research, asking other moms in the homeschooling community, and ultimately learning a lot about the life cycle of lice, I created an extremely effective solution that had wonderful side effects.

My remedy is a two-step process. The first part is shampooing daily with a shampoo infused with peppermint oil. You can use almost any shampoo and simply add some drops of peppermint essential oil to it. The strong mint is an irritant to the lice. The second part is combing your child's hair after each wash with a lice comb. The lice comb is really more important than the mint shampoo. Lice grow from egg to maturity in a 14-day period, so by combing out every egg and louse daily for 2 weeks, you can completely eliminate the entire population.

When my kids had lice growing up, we'd gather in our kitchen every evening for what became a 14-day ritual of pleasant smells, loving touch, and genuine conversation. I washed both Ryan's and Kimber's hair in the kitchen sink with the peppermint shampoo and then thoroughly combed out all the lice and eggs with the lice comb. Because I am very nearsighted, I needed Ryan to help me be sure I got all of Kimber's hair cleaned, and Kimber to ensure I got everything off Ryan's head. The kids were astonishingly cooperative because the social pressure had given them a strong desire to get through this. We laughed and joked a lot. I loved getting to wash and comb my kids' hair again, especially Ryan, who was becoming a boy's boy and not as interested in hugs and kisses from Mom as he used to be.

I am still amazed at the simplicity and effectiveness of it. What would have been a quick splash of noxious chemicals and social isolation instead became a time of togetherness, conversation, and devoted care. Rather than separating us, those head lice gave us the opportunity to grow closer. I still remember it fondly. Can you imagine that—fond memories involving head lice? But it's true. It was a powerful experience that we shared as a family.

As I've learned more and more about home medicine, I've realized that illnesses and injuries mark very special times for families. They show us how to rely on each other, encourage us to strengthen our empathy, and teach us to focus on what matters most—the health and well-being of those we love. You can bring this power and meaning to your own family, too.

Bringing Back the Power of Herbal Medicine

Before the invention of 24-hour drug stores and emergency rooms, herbal medicines and home remedies were the norm everywhere. Because so many people now rely on the authority of the medical establishment, the prevailing idea seems to be that home remedies are primitive, superstitious, and ineffective. But the opposite is true. Herbal medicines have been helping people avoid and recover from minor and major conditions throughout human history. They are powerful, and they have a much deeper connection with our spirit than something synthesized in a lab.

Don't think I'm totally against modern medicine. I regularly get all kinds of blood-work and other diagnostics done. And if I ever need major surgery, I'm certainly not going to try to perform it at home. My left leg was sliced open by a piece of sheet metal one Sunday morning, and you bet I am deeply appreciative of the morphine, the doctor, and the 22 stiches I had after that accident!

The medical system has a lot to offer when it comes to diagnostics and critical, acute care. But it has limitations, too. For one thing, it's expensive. The cost of health care and pharmaceuticals has skyrocketed, and it just keeps going up.

Hospitals also don't have the atmosphere of love and nurturing that you find at home. They're filled with beeping monitors, blinking lights, strange smells and noises, and constant interruptions by nurses coming in to check your vitals. This is not an atmosphere of healing. Sleep and good food—the two universals of healing—are impossible to get in a hospital. And although good doctors and nurses want to help you, they can never care as much about you as your spouse and kids can. They'll never have the same drive and single-minded focus on returning you to health as a family member would.

Going to the doctor can also be dangerous. If your only tool is a hammer, every problem starts to look like a nail. A doctor's main tools are drugs and surgery. If you come in with a problem, guess what they'll want to treat you with. Iatrogenic deaths, those caused by medical care, are the third leading cause of death in the United States. This can be from drug reactions, hospital-acquired infections, unnecessary surgeries, or medical errors. For those times that a hospital visit is unavoidable, you really need a family member with you, acting as your advocate, and watching out for your best interests.

It's time to move the center of healing for common ailments back to the home. This is where the modern medicine woman or man comes in. These healers take responsibility for their own health, and that of their families, by acquiring the basic skills and knowledge to treat common illness and injuries at home, naturally. You *can* gain this knowledge and experience, and this chapter explains the seven stages on this path. It's a journey you can continue your whole life, but it doesn't take years to start being useful. In fact, you can take the first step right now.

how old is herbal medicine?

In 1991, a German tourist discovered a man frozen in the ice of the Ötztal Alps. "Ötzi," as he came to be called, was dated to 3300 B.C.E. Among his possessions, Ötzi carried a medicine bag containing an antiparasitic, antibacterial birch fungus, likely used to treat a whipworm infestation he was suffering from. His stomach also contained the remains of an antiparasitic fern.

Analysis of Ötzi's body showed that he had recovered from various illnesses and injuries before ending up in the ice. He even had tattoo marks at traditional acupuncture points along his body. This evidence suggests that humans living at that time already had a well-developed understanding of the body's healing processes and herbal medicine.

Stage One: Your Declaration

It starts with intention. Intention is powerful, and a declaration sets that intention firmly in place. You can create real change by a making a single, firmly declared intention. Think of the United States. It came into being with the incredibly powerful Declaration of Independence.

It's as simple as saying . . .

"I declare that I will become a medicine woman [or medicine man]."

Once you make a declaration, you'll be amazed at the resources you've never noticed before that will come forward to help you achieve your goal. As Paulo Coelho writes in his book *The Alchemist*, "When you want something, all the universe conspires in helping you to achieve it."

Your journey will be filled with small steps, giant leaps, profound discoveries, and powerful moments. You'll also have a lot of mistakes and false starts. That's normal. Don't be discouraged. These, too, are parts of your story. We must all go through rough patches in order to fully learn. But eventually, the healer path will open a new world of health, freedom, and purpose. And it all starts with the power of a single declaration.

Stage Two: Your First Taste of Power

Years ago, when Ryan was a little baby, I had mastitis, which is a breast infection. I was having those high and fast spikes in fever, and my breast was red and sore. I didn't think too much about it, maybe because I was in that breastfeeding stupor that happens to women. But Dave, my husband, got deeply concerned. Overly concerned in my opinion. I mean, it was just a little infection. But as I soon learned, he had very good reason to be fearful.

As a young boy growing up in rural South Texas, Dave earned his spending money by milking the family cow and selling the excess. His cow got mastitis in one of her udders and ultimately died of the infection. He saw how a small infection can kill a very large animal fairly quickly. And in this case, it was an expensive animal that he depended on for his income, and he had firsthand experience of the danger and consequences of what could happen.

Fortunately, we had a midwife who had a lot of experience with breast infections and how to treat them naturally. Our midwife showed Dave how to make a poultice out of a cabbage. He set aside the big outer leaves and then cut up the rest of the cabbage into pieces, just like you would for coleslaw. I think he also might have chopped in a small amount of ginger and a few other plant materials, but the bulk of it was cabbage. Then, using the big outer leaves to hold it all together, we completely covered the swollen and sore breast with the chopped cabbage poultice. We kept the poultice on for several hours before changing it out for a fresh one and then did this a few more times over the next night and day. It astonished both of us how effective this treatment was. The infection cleared up completely in less than 2 days.

When you successfully treat an ailment for the first time, it will change you forever. It's amazing to realize that you really have the power to heal yourself and your family. You may feel a buzz of excitement, a sense of awed wonder, or something completely different. Whatever it is, take a moment to savor the experience and be grateful for this stage of your journey.

Most of us have minor ailments that seem to recur in our lives, and we have experience with how long it takes for them to heal using our regular techniques. Ailments such as these are great ones to start trying to treat with herbal remedies. It should be a health issue that is not super critical and that you already have some experience with. In other words, definitely start small, and don't try to cure cancer with your first attempt.

For example, we've had several cases of fractured or contused ribs in my family. We are a very sporty, outdoorsy, rough-and-tumble bunch, and we frequently come back from vacations bruised, sprained, and physically exhausted from all the tubing, rock climbing, skiing, hiking, running, zip lining, and whatever other outdoor adventures we find. Both Dave and I have busted our ribs multiple times over the years. It is an injury we are familiar with. There really isn't much conventional medicine can do except offer painkillers. We know we're in for approximately 6 to 8 weeks of pain and being careful not to take deep breaths or laugh too hard.

My last rib injury was from a skateboarding accident a few years ago. Our chiropractor confirmed with x-rays that my rib was not broken, but it was very badly contused and had a minor fracture. Instead of the usual wait-and-be-careful method of healing, I decided this time to try treating the injury with herbals. I used a combination of an external prickly pear poultice and an arnica liniment, and I also took herbal infusions made with comfrey and nettles. The rib healed in 3 weeks, which is about half of the normal time.

Stage Three: The Eight Preparations

There are eight basic ways to prepare herbs for use as medicine. The simplest is to use the raw plant as you find it growing in your yard. But because bark and roots often are not so easy to work with and take directly, medicine-making requires putting the healing ingredients into other forms, like lotions or pills, to make them easier to apply or ingest. There are also many times when the fresh plant isn't available, so methods such as tincturing preserve the medicinal qualities of the plant. Some of the preparations, like syrups and jellies, are best when you have to get medicine into children (or reluctant spouses who are acting like children). These different methods optimize our ability to naturally use plants as medicines.

Here are the eight basic preparations:

1. Fresh plants
2. Pills
3. Teas and infusions
4. Tinctures
5. Liniments and wound sprays
6. Lotions and salves
7. Syrups and gelatins
8. Poultices

I go into depth on how to make each of the eight preparations in the next chapter.

Stage three usually comes without a lot of pomp and circumstance, and it doesn't make itself known with one shining example of herbal achievement. You just gradually realize that you've been learning your way around the herbs and home medicines and you are becoming more comfortable with them. In this stage, your skills are growing, and you're on your way to gaining even more confidence and ability.

Stage Four: 12 Common Ailments

You are now at the level where you can handle the most common illnesses and injuries that come up in everyday life. You've seen ailments come and go, and you know you can handle them without making a late-night run to the pharmacy or emergency room. The fear and uncertainty have disappeared, replaced with courage and capability.

You have several good books on herbalism and home medicine that you refer to regularly (and there are a lot of good ones out there!). Your library of herb books includes quite a few that are specific to your region, and you are getting good at identifying what grows locally. Your pantry has a small collection of home medicines you've made and use frequently. And you've started developing a network of trusted healers, growers, and other medicine-makers.

You are also well aware that you do have limits, and you know roughly where those limits are.

But by this point, you can confidently treat at least 12 common ailments that come up frequently in your family. Each family is a little different (not everyone busts their ribs!), but to get you started, here is a list of the everyday health issues most families typically deal with:

1. Burns
2. Cuts and wounds
3. Nose, eye, and other mucosal problems
4. Fever
5. Indigestion and stomachache
6. Anxiety
7. Insomnia
8. Muscle aches and pains
9. Topical infections
10. Bites, stings, and rashes
11. Coughs and sore throats
12. Headaches

I do a lot of radio and television interviews, and sometimes people will call in asking about either some severe medical condition or a specific unusual plant. I am only a home medicine-maker; I am not a trained professional herbalist. I learn about and work with plant medicines in my spare time, and I focus on what I need to know to help my family most. I'm happy knowing I can handle the most common, minor health conditions we experience, but I know I have limits. I would be way out of my league if I tried to treat a major disease or a severe injury. Other people have dedicated their lives to understanding herbal medicine more deeply, and I am delighted to have developed friendships with them so I can reach out to them when necessary. At this stage, you should be empowered by what you know, but you should also have a very clear understanding of what you don't know and where your own limits are.

A reassuring bit of news is that you do not need an encyclopedia's worth of plant knowledge to be able to reach this stage in your home medicine journey. You only really need to know the properties of about 5 to 10 plants to be able to handle most of the minor needs that come up in a family. Many herbs have several different uses. For example, the prickly pear is a great poulticing material for wounds and sprains. It is also good for treating burns and stings. The fruits and pads are edible, and the flowers are quite tasty, too.

Although prickly pear does grow everywhere, it is happiest in the desert Southwest. In your region, common plantain might be one of your most abundant favorites. The young plantain leaves in the spring are edible, as are the seeds. The older leaves make great poulticing material, either fresh or rehydrated from dried.

I highly recommend that you explore the medicinal properties of the herbs that grow locally in your yard or area. Preferably it's a plant that is considered "weedy," in that it is abundant and your harvesting it won't affect the population. Start with one, learn about it, and use it at least several times in different ways. Then pick another herb friend. Start slowly and allow this process to unfold naturally. One day you'll realize you have a good knowledge base and can confidently handle at least a dozen common ailments.

the five great herbs

If you want to send an herbalist into spasms, ask him or her what their favorite herb is. There are so many great plants to work with, it's really tough to choose just one, let alone the "top five," but I've got some suggestions here for you to start with. I've chosen these because they grow easily almost everywhere, are commonly available commercially, and each has multiple uses. In fact, these five have so many more uses than the brief descriptions I've included here. If you just made a new human friend, you would not expect to know the complexity of their life in just a 5-minute conversation, but those first 5 minutes would give you a good idea of whether you wanted to pursue a deeper relationship. Consider this a short flirting session to see if you want to get to know these herbs better.

Chamomile. Chamomile has been used medicinally for centuries. The most common way to use chamomile is to prepare a tea from the dried flowers. Chamomile is a "nervine," which means it is very soothing to your nervous system. Chamomile tea helps you calm down and relax at the end of a hectic day or any stressful time. The German chamomile (*Matricaria chamomilla*) is an annual plant, and the Roman chamomile (*Chamaemelum nobile*) is a perennial. Medicinally they are essentially the same. Chamomile has anti-inflammatory properties, which help reduce muscle spasms and hay fever. Chamomile also helps heal and restore the kidneys. Your adrenal glands sit on top of your kidneys, and the two are intimately related. If you have a tendency toward adrenal fatigue, drinking chamomile tea daily will help.

Comfrey leaf. Comfrey leaf is great to use in a poultice to treat wounds, lacerations, broken bones, or sprains. Comfrey's botanical name is *Symphytum officinale*. "Symphytum" means "bones growing together," and the common name for comfrey is "knitbone." It actually will heal bones and cause them to knit back together. Comfrey contains a chemical called allantoin, which has two really great properties. It's really penetrating, so you can put a comfrey poultice on a broken bone, even if the skin's not broken, and the allantoin will soak through the tissue and get to the bones. It's also a deeply nourishing tonic if you make an infusion to extract the nutrients out of the leaves and drink it.

Mallow. You probably have mallow (*Malva neglecta*) growing in your lawn right now. Mallow has two cousins, marshmallow (*Althaea officinalis*) and hollyhocks (*Alcea rosea*), which have similar medicinal properties. The whole plant is medicinal—leaves, roots, flowers, and seedpods—and contains a lot of mucilage, which makes it very soothing. Mallow is really great for bronchitis, bladder inflammations, or bladder infections. Basically, for anything wrong with your gastrointestinal tract, mallow is just fantastic.

What I love most about mallow is that the whole plant is edible. After the flowers are done, the plant makes this little round seed package that looks like a little tiny green cheese wheel. That's my favorite part. You can eat the little cheese wheels at all stages, from green to when the seeds are crunchy mature.

Cayenne pepper. Cayenne pepper (*Capsicum annuum*) is great when you have a crisis situation. My friend Dr. Patrick Jones says that in his veterinary practice, he has saved more animal lives with cayenne than with all the other herbs combined. He has used it to treat dogs hit by cars. The dog can be bleeding from the nose and the mouth, his gums are white, his eyes are rolled back in his head, and he's not very responsive. After a squirt of cayenne tincture in his mouth, the dog will come back as though a switch has been turned on. His gums turn pink, he is alert, his breathing is better, and his heart rate improves. Cayenne is a premier crisis herb that is great for shock, blood loss, and even heart attack. The dried, powdered form of cayenne (yes, the stuff you can buy at the grocery store) applied topically to a gushing wound will stop bleeding. Even if the first coating of cayenne gets pushed out by the blood, keep applying more, and it will soon stop.

Echinacea. Echinacea is one of the most popular herbs to tincture, and for good reason. It's great for systemic bacterial infections, sepsis, or anytime you need to support the immune system. People often take echinacea for colds and flus, which are viral infections, and although the echinacea will probably help in that situation, it really is better for bacterial infections. If I have a large wound or burn, in addition to topical treatments, I take echinacea to prevent infection internally. Echinacea is helpful for cartilage injuries, too, because it stimulates hyaluronic acid production, which is mostly what your cartilage is made out of. If you have a torn rotator cuff or similar injury, echinacea can help.

Purple and yellow coneflowers, the common names for two echinacea genus plants, are very popular ornamentals and may be in your flower garden right now. Both are good for making medicine. The roots have the most medicine, but tinctures made from the flowers are plenty strong for most common home needs and are so much easier to harvest. The best medicinal species to grow at home is *Echinacea purpurea*.

Stage Five: You Use Herbal Medicine Proactively

When he was young, my son, Ryan, once asked me, "Hey, Mommy, you know how when you are asleep and you wake up? Well, when you are awake, can you wake up even more?" Of course, the answer is yes. When you reach this stage of home medicine-making, you understand that plant medicines not only heal injuries and common ailments but powerfully boost your health when you are well, too.

This stage marks a turning point. You can use plants to react to health problems, but you can also use them to stop illnesses before they start. I admit you won't really be able to stop all injuries and illnesses. But if you take steps to actively promote robust health and well-being, you will prevent a lot of them. For example, well-cared-for joints are less likely to become sprained or develop arthritis. A well-nourished, vitalized immune system is less likely to be caught off guard by a cold, flu, or virus. And when an accident or illness does manage to sneak through, you'll be in better shape to heal and recover.

You can use herbs proactively to keep nudging yourself toward greater and greater health, continually making small shifts in your system toward health. This may take the form of nutritional vinegars, nourishing infusions, and immune-supporting tonics. Or you may be experimenting with spices. Indigenous peoples had the traditional wisdom to spice their foods not only for flavor but also for the nutritional benefits. Many of our kitchen spices, such as anise, mint, sage, thyme, fennel, ginger, and rosemary, are known as carminatives and help with digestion, provide micronutrients, and increase gut biodiversity.

You can learn how to proactively prepare your body for the changes in the seasons. For example, at the end of winter and into early spring, you can use fresh greens in different preparations to help clean and tonify your blood and lymph. In the summer, you can add foods and herbs such as mallow and cucumber that moisturize and cool. In the autumn, maybe you make batches of fire cider and elderberry syrup because you know cold and flu season is right around the corner. Before meals at any time of year, but especially before a big holiday meal feast, perhaps you nibble on a dandelion leaf. The slightly bitter taste is an excellent digestive aid prior to eating.

fire cider: winter sickness prevention

I am not a big fan of overly spicy foods, yet every autumn I make a batch of the incredibly spicy "fire cider," and I am continually amazed how much I love it. It seems like my body knows it wants this support and adjusts my tastes accordingly.

Fire cider prepares my body for all those wonderful events during the holidays, when I am eating heavy and rich foods I wouldn't normally touch and hanging out with relatives who have come in from everywhere (and brought their airplane germs with them), and we pack tightly into rooms that do not have anywhere near the ventilation needed for that many people. It's a recipe for passing colds and flu! But now that I make fire cider in early November, I never get sick over the holidays anymore.

To make fire cider, you chop up and combine a bunch of different antibacterial and antimicrobial plants. For example, combine ½ cup each of garlic cloves, ginger root, and horseradish root to form a great base and then add whatever else you have on hand, such as juniper berries, hot peppers, onions, turmeric, and more. Nature is not super precise, and you don't need to be either. You chop the components into pieces about the size of corn kernels, stuff them into a quart-sized canning jar, and fill the jar to the top with the best-quality apple cider vinegar you can find. Use a plastic lid on the jar because vinegar tends to corrode metal lids. Shake it a bit every day for the first few days and then let it finish on the counter or in the pantry for another 2 weeks or so. Strain off and bottle the spicy liquid, and add the solids to your compost pile.

I splash fire cider on salads, use it to make ceviche, put it in chilis, add it to guacamole, or just take a tablespoon straight. Check out the fabulous fire cider recipes gathered by Rosemary Gladstar in her book *Fire Cider! 101 Zesty Recipes for Health-Boosting Remedies Made with Apple Cider Vinegar.*

At this stage, as you've been proactively incorporating more and more plant medicines into your lifestyle, friends and coworkers may notice that you also get sick less frequently. When you do get sick, it's usually mild and you recover quickly. They also might comment on how much clearer your skin is or how beautiful your hair and nails look. Things only get better as we go further.

Stage Six: You Grow or Wild Tend Your Own Medicines

In the beginning, it's easiest to buy herbs locally or order them online. That's a great way to start! But by now, you are discovering the increased potency of homegrown and wild tended herbs. Just like the food in your garden, the herbs you grow and wild tend will be more powerful than those you buy. One reason is because, like your garden plants, these medicinal plants will have adapted to the local environment and will be especially suited to live in it. It is astonishing how many times people discover that the medicine they need just happens to be a "weed" growing in their yard. Another reason is freshness and purity. Most commercially grown herbs sit in shipping containers for weeks as they travel halfway across the world to reach your grocery store, not to mention that these containers are then usually fumigated and irradiated. When you grow your herbs yourself, you can harvest them at the peak of their potency and process them immediately. They are truly living medicines.

As your skill grows and you watch the cycles of the plants, you'll learn what growing conditions each plant likes best. You'll discover which parts of the plant are most powerful, and you'll be able to tell exactly when they are ready to be harvested. You'll even learn to select between two plants of the same species to tweak your medicines for maximum efficacy.

plant name fun fact

When a plant species name ends in "officinale," that's an indication the plant has a long history of being used as an herbal medicine. For example, comfrey is *Symphytum officinale*, dandelion is *Taraxacum officinale*, and calendula is *Calendula officinalis*.

The officinale tag means "from the officina," which was the little room in the monastery where the monks kept the medicinal plants. So plants with those names have been in use for hundreds of years.

Just like with your own homegrown food, there is something magical about the connection you build with plants as you tend to them and care for them. The taste of the food you grow yourself is superb beyond anything you can buy, and similarly, the medicines you grow or wildcraft yourself can have potency beyond anything that can be purchased.

One of my trusted health-care providers, Nicole Telkes, is also the founder of the Wildflower School of Botanical Medicine. Like many fine herbalists, Nikki regularly offers free plant walks to the community. Nikki is a bioregional herbalist in that she focuses solely on teaching people how to make medicines out of the weeds that grow in their yards or neighborhoods. Nikki told me that the reason she offers the free plant walks is that when people realize valuable medicine is growing in their local greenbelts or parks, they have a different relationship to the land and begin to care for and defend it. The benefits for the environment are also powerful.

Stage Seven: Plants Speak to You

Nature is not a linear process. For many people, this stage takes many years to cultivate, but for others, it's the calling of plants that first gets them excited about herbal medicine.

We form connections with plants, just like we do with animals and people. Although plant communication is subtler than a barking dog or a chatty neighbor, you can become familiar enough and open enough to hear the plants "speaking" to you. Essentially, it's about intuition and developing your connections to the world around you. Do I mean that you will actually hear voices talking to you? Stay with me here. That's not necessarily the case, although for some people this does happen.

Here's a more common experience. When you have a strong connection to plants, you might wake up feeling sick one morning and notice a pull or "calling" from a certain jar of herbs in your pantry. Dr. Patrick Jones, founder of the HomeGrown School of Herbalism, says his jars of herbs sometimes practically jump off the shelf at him. Or maybe you will have a craving for elderberries one day and decide to make an elderberry tea or take a swig of some elderberry syrup you have on hand. Later, you realize that the rest of your family is coming down with a sore throat or cold and you aren't. Maybe it's a coincidence, but from the thousands of people who have told me of this kind of experience, I don't think so.

Sometimes you might be walking in the park and suddenly one plant just seems to glow more brightly than the others, almost asking you to pay attention to it. Sit down and hang out with that plant. Quiet your mind and open yourself to images, feelings, sensations, or quiet knowing. Or maybe nothing at all. But see if you can identify the plant, perhaps sketch it, or take some photos, and then go research it. If nothing else, you'll be learning a little bit more about one of your neighbors.

Just a few days ago, I was walking through the woods and literally had a plant grab me. Its thorny, sprawling branches hooked into the sleeve of my shirt and demanded I stop. Turns out, the plant was a wild rose bush and was loaded with perfectly dried rose hips. I was delighted for the interruption in my walk and collected a bunch of rose hips. I used them in teas and made some homemade vitamin C pills for when I travel. (You learn how to make your own pills in Chapter 8.)

Another technique to try is passing your hand slowly over your different living plants or herbal preparations and see if any seem to be pulling you forward.

One of the easiest and most direct ways to connect with a plant is by simply offering your breath. I love to smell a flower or a group of leaves. Then I cup the flower or leaves with my hands, focus my breath on that area, and then smell again. Some plants just love this and after my exhale respond immediately with a much richer aroma. Not all plants respond this way, but finding the ones that do is a super fun thing to do with kids.

Go slowly and really listen to yourself and the plants. Don't worry if nothing happens at first. Relationships are built, not forced. You currently may have belief systems that prevent you from experiencing this aspect of reality. Keep at it. Given time, the answers will come to you faster and more frequently.

Accessing knowledge beyond your normal five senses is a skill anyone can develop and is extremely useful in so many other areas of your life. Working with the plant kingdom is a great way to begin to learn this. At this stage, you have had direct, first-hand experience with that greater wisdom, and a whole new world is opening to you.

Getting Started with Garlic

Now that you can see the full potential of plant medicine, let's get started with garlic, an ingredient that is easy to incorporate into your life and will give you an overall health boost. Many trained herbalists suggest using garlic as a "starter medicine." Like almost all the herbal remedies I mention in this book, garlic has a long history as a health remedy and has been used for hundreds and thousands of years. Specifically, garlic is thought to have properties that are antibiotic, antifungal, and antiviral. The father of modern medicine, Hippocrates, who lived around 400 B.C.E., used garlic to treat wounds, fight infections, and ease digestive disorders.

If you think about it, those ancient Roman and Greek warriors should have had a lot more health problems. They spent their lives stabbing each other with swords and lances, and when they weren't doing that, they were getting shot with arrows. Yes, some of them died from their wounds, but a lot of them lived. That means the medics who lived in those times used powerful herbal antibiotics. Garlic was definitely one of them. According to Stephen Buhner, a modern expert and author of several excellent books on herbal antibiotics, "If only one herb could be used to combat an epidemic spread of antibiotic-resistant bacteria, [garlic] would be it."

Yes, that bulb of garlic you probably have in your kitchen right now (scientific name *Allium sativum*) is actually a powerful medicine. And best of all, it does not create the same problems of antibiotic resistance like its commercially produced (distant) cousins. Its ability to avoid antibiotic resistance lies in its complexity. Garlic naturally contains 33 sulfur compounds, 17 amino acids, and multiple other components. Most of garlic's therapeutic benefits come from a sulfur compound called allicin, which gives garlic its microbial properties.

Interestingly, raw garlic does not contain allicin, but it does contain two ingredients that create allicin when they come in contact: alliin, a sulfur-rich amino acid, and alliinase, a protein-based enzyme. These two compounds are physically separated in the whole clove, but when garlic is crushed, minced, or otherwise broken, the physical barrier is removed, and the alliinase enzyme begins to convert alliin into allicin.

How to Use Garlic Medicinally

I use garlic as a remedy for many health issues. I take it as a preventative when I feel like I'm on the verge of a sickness or about to head into a stressful time and my body will be run down. I also use it to fight infections. If I have a wound I'm worried about, I take garlic internally to help prevent infection. I also make a soothing garlic oil to treat earaches.

Be sure the garlic bulbs you get are fresh. The cloves should be firm and pungent. If they're dry, soft, or mushy, or if they have darkened brown or black spots, the garlic is old. Old garlic does not have the potency you want.

Also, for medicinal purposes, it's best to eat garlic raw. I certainly love the taste of garlic in my vegetable stir-fries, but cooking destroys or weakens a lot of garlic's most active ingredients, especially the allicin. Also, in pill or powder form, the allicin just doesn't survive the processing process. The potency you are looking for is only available in fresh, vibrant garlic.

Here is how to prepare the garlic:

1. Start with a clove taken from a good-quality bulb.

2. Peel the clove.

3. Use either a garlic press or a knife to chop the clove. If you are using a knife, first crush the clove on a chopping board with the flat side of the knife and then finely mince the crushed clove.

4. After cutting, wait at least a minute for the alliin to be converted to allicin. You might even want to wait a little longer. Research indicates that allowing chopped or crushed garlic to sit for 10 minutes before using it significantly increases the amount of allicin produced. I wouldn't let it sit for much longer than that, though, because allicin is a volatile molecule that quickly starts to break down into other compounds.

5. Eat the crushed clove. I eat it straight, but you can juice it with other vegetables or take the crushed or minced garlic with a spoonful of melted butter or coconut oil. I'd just caution you to avoid taking it with simple sugars or starchy carbohydrates because these feed infection. Also, be sure to eat the garlic with something else in your stomach. It is powerful medicine, and eating raw garlic on an empty stomach can lead to nausea, heartburn, or worse.

How Much Garlic Should You Take?

Be sure to take more than one clove a day. One clove won't be enough because garlic affects the body more slowly than other medicines, and you need a greater amount to reap the benefits. If I am using garlic as a preventative, I eat a clove every 3 or 4 hours for a total of about three cloves a day. If I am fighting a more serious infection, I increase that dosage to six or nine cloves a day. Some people have reported taking even higher dosages, but go slow at first, and again, be sure to eat garlic with something in your stomach.

How Long Should You Follow a Garlic Regimen?

Healing with garlic is a multiday process. Keep checking in with yourself. After one day, how are you progressing? Are you better or worse? Do you need to adjust your dosages up or down? After two days, are you seeing some improvements? Remember to be sure you are eating a good diet and getting enough sleep. Garlic can't do everything on its own; you have to help the process of healing. Anytime you are ill or feeling on the verge of sickness, it is vital that you nourish your body with good food and be sure to rest. Focus on ingesting fresh vegetables, fruits, probiotic foods, healthy oils, high-quality meats, and plenty of water. As I mentioned earlier, you should avoid eating infection-feeding foods such as simple sugars and starchy carbs.

Usually by the third day, you'll know how well it is working for you. And as with many herbal medicines, it's a good idea to continue to take it for a period after your symptoms are gone. Just because you are feeling better doesn't mean your body is done healing. Continue taking garlic for an extra day or two to help your immune system complete its job.

Although garlic is very powerful medicine and can heal many things, it certainly doesn't cure everything. If you are not seeing any improvement after a week, it is probably time to go see a health-care provider.

garlic and earaches

I'm prone to earaches that result from lake water going up into my ears after I've crashed off my skis, and I've found that garlic is very helpful for curing them. For earaches, garlic should be taken both internally (as described earlier) and topically in the form of a simple-to-make ear oil.

To make the ear oil, simply prepare your raw clove as described on page 149. Then, add a few pieces of chopped garlic in a small pot with about 1 or 2 teaspoons of a good oil, such as olive oil or coconut oil. Gently warm—but don't overheat—the oil and garlic for a few minutes to let the garlic infuse. Then use an eyedropper to drip the warm, soothing garlic oil into your ear.

It feels so nice! And, even better, you've got the antiviral, antibiotic, and antifungal properties of garlic helping heal your ear.

....

Garlic Side Effects

There is some debate about whether garlic, with its antibiotic properties, also kills off your gut flora. Some studies seem to show that it spares certain types of beneficial gut bacteria and even, with its prebiotic qualities, nourishes them. Others indicate that garlic does, indeed, inhibit the growth of friendly bacteria. As unsettled as this question is, when taking garlic, I'd suggest also proactively planning to restore your gut flora as if you had been taking pharmaceutical antibiotics.

You can do this by eating fermented and cultured foods while you are following a course of garlic and immediately thereafter. Fermented veggies, sauerkraut, kefir, and kombucha are just a few whole foods that provide probiotics to boost your gut health.

Garlic is also contraindicated with certain medications, such as birth control pills, nonsteroidal anti-inflammatory drugs (NSAIDs), and some drugs used to treat HIV infections. So if you are taking any of these drugs, please talk with a trusted health-care provider before starting a course of garlic. Also, because garlic acts as a blood thinner, it can increase the risk of bleeding. If you take an anticoagulant such as warfarin or are about to undergo surgery, proceed very cautiously.

The more common physical side effects of eating garlic are what you'd expect—bad breath, body odor, bloating, and upset stomach. But in my experience, eating fresh, raw garlic does not create as strong breath and body odor as eating cooked garlic does. My solution? If anyone is annoyed, simply feed them some garlic, too.

And there you go—your first home medicine! Garlic is really an amazing herb and a great ally.

Health in the Home

No matter at what stage you are, you can start moving the center of healing back to the home. It's a very simple and satisfying form of richness. So much love and trust is generated with making, using, and sharing home medicines. And as you do, you'll be generating true wealth.

chapter summary

- Caring for your family's common health needs builds love, trust, and real wealth.

- The seven stages of becoming a home medicine-maker are as follows:

  - Declaration. You declare your intention to become a medicine woman or man.

  - First taste of power. You have successfully used a plant medicine and experienced the healing power.

  - The eight basic preparations. You have worked with fresh plants, made tinctures, created salves, and more.

  - The 12 common ailments. You can handle most of the 12 common illnesses and injuries that come up.

  - You use herbal medicines proactively. You head off problems before they start.

  - You grow or wildcraft your own medicines. You increase the potency of your medicines by getting closer to your plants.

  - Plants speak to you. Your intuition and sense of connectedness with plants and healing are strong.

additional resources

For more information on herbal medicine, check out these websites:

- www.GarlicMiracles.com. A free, detailed ebook with more in-depth info on how to use garlic as your first home medicine.

- www.HomemadeFireCider.com. A short video in which I show you step-by-step how I make my fire cider each November.

- www.MakeYourOwnMedicine.com. A free introductory training video on how to start making your own medicine. In the fourth part of this short series, I break open my own homemade first-aid kit and show you how I prepare for many of the minor medical issues that come up in my family.

- www.HomeMedicine101.com. An online training that explains how to treat the 12 most common ailments that come up in a family. The training offers a variety of herbs for each ailment to ensure you'll be able to find something that grows locally in your area.

- www.MarjoryWildHerbs.com. A store where I have limited quantities of extremely high-quality herbs grown by farmers I know and trust. My business model is to go out of business. My goal is to get so many medicinal herbs growing locally that it doesn't make sense to sell them anymore. So to purchase any of these extremely high-quality herbs, you must make a commitment to grow an herb yourself, too.

chapter 8

the preparations: eight types of medicine, from pills to poultices, and **how to make them**

There is one thing I know about your great-grandmother. She didn't have a Cuisinart, a blender, or a microwave.

Throughout history, herbal preparations have been made by people who had very primitive resources. They cooked on wood-burning stoves or open hearths. Perhaps they had a few utensils, a chopping board, and bowls but no specialized tools, no kitchen gadgets, no electricity, no gas stoves where they could adjust a flame with a knob. In many cases, a pounding rock and smooth surface were the only implements available.

And this is good news. Basically, it means that making medicine is very simple and easy. If they did it back then, with so few helpers, for sure you can do it now.

Some preparations are super simple—as simple as picking and eating a fresh dandelion leaf. Others have a few more steps involved. But none of them are complicated, and all of them will be invaluable in helping you and your family overcome the common illnesses and injuries of life.

Whenever possible, speak kindly to the medicines as you make them. Say encouraging words. Sing songs. Send positive energy. I know some of you will think this is silly, but I've seen others test this and have witnessed it myself in my own medicines. Your energy and intentions will amplify the effects of your medicines. Try it. You'll be surprised at the power in your words and intentions.

The most important thing to remember is *the plant is the medicine*. Not the preparation. We make and use preparations for convenience. It's a lot easier to take a dropperful of a tincture than it is to try to get the medicinal qualities out of a tough root directly. Making a salve is a much nicer way to apply the soothing qualities of calendula to your skin than trying to rub the flowers on your face. Making a syrup is a fantastic way to get more herbs into kids.

Always keep in mind that the medicine is in the plant. That leads us to our first preparation.

Fresh

This is as simple as it gets. Just pick a leaf, pop it in your mouth, and eat it. Herbal medicine doesn't have to be fancy. Remember, we're not really *making* medicines. The plants made the medicine, and we're just moving those medicines around into convenient applications. Chewing on a leaf is every bit as much herbal medicine as making a pill or a tincture.

There is a tragic story of an early American homesteading family who lost a member to scurvy. They buried him under a big pine tree. The tragedy is that scurvy is a disease of malnutrition brought on by a lack of vitamin C, and the needles of pine trees (*Pinus* sp.) are a rich source of vitamin C.

Chewing on some pine needles is about as simple as it gets. Vitamin C, or ascorbic acid, is destroyed by heat, so rather than make a tea of them, the best way to absorb pine needles' vitamins is to simply chew the needles raw. The older needles contain more vitamin C but also taste more "piney."

A U.S. Department of Agriculture (USDA) Forest Service study showed that 1 gram of eastern white pine needles contained between 0.72 and 1.87 milligrams (mg) ascorbic acid (vitamin C). If you are used to grabbing a bottle of 1,000 mg vitamin C pills off the shelf in the supermarket supplements aisle, you might scoff at that teeny little 1 mg of vitamin C in a few pine needles. But there is a world of difference between whole foods and lab-created supplements. For example, numerous studies have shown that the tiny 5 mg of vitamin C in a fresh, medium-sized apple have more antioxidant activity in the human body than 1,500 mg of ascorbic acid contained in a pill.

The easiest way to "eat" pine needles is to chew them, let your saliva mix with the plant's juices, swallow the liquid, and spit out the pulp. When do you ever get to spit anymore? Just maybe don't do it around your in-laws. If you're like me, they already think you are weird enough.

healing with fresh herbs

In addition to chewing pine needles to boost your vitamin C, here are some other ailments you can try to address using fresh herbs:

- **To relieve headaches and other aches and pains. Chew the young, green twigs of aspen (*Populus* sp.), willow (*Salix* sp.), or poplar (*Populus* sp.). The active ingredient in the willow bark, salicin, is a mild pain reliever and a good alternative to aspirin.**

- **To freshen your mouth and your brain. Fresh peppermint (*Mentha × piperita*) and rosemary (*Rosemarinus officinalis*) leaves can freshen a stale mouth and stimulate clear thinking and sharper memory. Drop a fresh sprig into your water bottle to add some zing to your water intake.**

- **To soothe the itch from small insect bites. Grab a leaf or two of plantain (*Plantago* sp.), chew, and use the mash as a small quantity of poultice to soothe the bite.**

- **To relieve indigestion. Try eating a dandelion leaf before meals.**

Fresh herbs do have a few limitations. Depending on the herb in question, they aren't always available year-round. Some herbs are too tough or too foul-tasting to use as is. Not everyone wants to gnaw on a piece of tree root. And in an emergency, having medicine prepared ahead of time can be invaluable because time can be a critical factor.

But as far as simplicity goes, nothing beats chewing a fresh herb.

Pills

You may think pills are the domain of pharmacies, and that medicine women and men are limited to strange, bubbling concoctions. We can make those bubbling concoctions, but a pill is a lot easier to carry with you when you travel.

Pills are also really simple to make. All you need is the medicinal herb of your choice, a binder herb, and a little water. That's it! The medicinal herb has the curative effect you're trying to achieve, and the binder holds everything together.

Slippery elm bark (*Ulmus rubra*) is a good binder for most pill preparations. Note that the slippery elm harvested from eastern forests is under a lot of pressure from overharvesting, but many other varieties of elm have the same properties. One example is the Chinese elm (*Ulmus parvifolia*). It is considered a "junk" tree in western states, but it has the same medicinal properties as the eastern species. If you have an elm tree in your yard, you might try it out yourself. All elm trees have this mucilaginous property. If you skin the bark from the young, new branches and then chew on a bit of the bark, you'll start to get some mucilaginous action—also known as slippery gluey slime. Once you've tried it, you can skin more young bark, dry it, and have it on hand for pill-making.

If you can't find a local or other alternative to the eastern elm, you can use other binders. I recommend marshmallow root (*Althaea officinalis*) or okra (*Abelmoschus esculentus*). Okra is in the same family as mallow, and both produce a lot of the mucilage that can bind pills together. Just slice an okra pod, dehydrate it, powder it, and use it in place of the suggested binder.

Now that you've got your binder, let's get to the medicine. You can make herbal pills out of a wide variety of different herbs. Pretty much anything you can powder (and that isn't toxic) can be made into an herbal pill. Because the convenience of pills makes them an excellent choice for travel, for your first attempt at pill-making, ask yourself what you might need when you're on the road. Immune boosters are a great choice.

Herbal pills are also a great vehicle for taking bad-tasting herbs. Just pop them in and swallow them before you have a chance to taste them. Many of the elders in the herbal community—and these are vibrant, alert, spry octogenarians—strongly recommend taking a small daily dose of gotu kola (*Centella asiatica*) to help with memory and ashwagandha (*Withania somnifera*) for stamina and strength. The problem is, these herbs taste really awful. The only way I can get myself to take them is in herbal pill form.

Making Herbal Pills

To make an herbal pill, you start by processing dried herbs into a powder. To do this, you can either grind the dried herbs with a mortar and pestle or pop them in your blender. I am a huge fan of using a coffee grinder for this purpose.

Combine roughly 80 percent of your medicinal herb and approximately 20 percent of your binder herb in a bowl. Stir in just a little bit of water at a time until the mixture reaches the consistency of Play-Doh. You want it moldable.

In our modern age, when a misplaced dot or an extra letter will send your computer into spasms of 404 errors, we have a tendency to want everything to be precise. Joseph Campbell, author of the book *The Hero with a Thousand Faces*, compared our computers to an Old Testament God who smote you down for the tiniest infraction of the rules. Nature is much more forgiving. If you want to try 90 percent medicinal herb to 10 percent binder, or perhaps you only have 70 percent and 30 percent, give those a try. The binder herbs also have gentle medicinal properties and tend to have a bit of sweetness. There weren't a lot of measuring cups around when these herbs were used in antiquity.

After you have mixed in enough water to make your herb dough, use your fingers to pinch off some of the dough and then roll up little pills in your hands. You could also roll the dough into a rope and use a knife to slice it into pills. Don't make the pills too big. Remember to keep them the size you are able to easily swallow.

Place your pills on a sheet of wax paper to dry. You can speed up the process by setting them in a food dehydrator on the lowest heat setting or in your oven on warm. Remember that heat often destroys medicinal properties, so go easy. Be sure your pills are well dried, or they will mold.

Store your dried pills in a tin or other airtight container. If kept away from moisture, extreme heat, or prolonged sunlight, your herbal pills should stay good for around a year.

Pill Tips

- If you accidentally add too much water, all is not lost. Just add more powdered herbs until the mixture returns to the desired consistency.

- Don't make your pills any larger than you want to swallow. It's a common mistake.

- Dry your pills thoroughly before storing them so they won't mold.

- Herbal pills have a 1-year shelf life, but they won't last as long if you started with older herbs. For maximum potency and shelf life, use the freshest herbs possible.

Teas

The humble cup of tea is an incredibly potent medicine. In wilderness survival schools, it is common knowledge that if you have the skills to make a cup of tea, you can pretty much survive anything. Plus, sitting down with a good friend and drinking a cup of tea can be powerfully healing, regardless of the herbs you are drinking.

Teas and infusions are both water-based extractions of an herb. Technically, a drink is only a tea if it contains leaves of the tea plant (*Camellia sinensis*). From this perspective, all other herbal "teas" are really herbal infusions. However, we're going to take the more casual (and accessible) approach and use these terms interchangeably.

A very rough distinction between teas and infusions has to do with how much herb you are using relative to the amount of water. In general, a tea involves a small amount of herb, say between 1 teaspoon and 1 tablespoon, to 1 cup of water. Infusions, on the other hand, use a much larger amount of herb, such as 1 cup of herb to 2 cups of water. Infusions can act as a powerful daily "multivitamin" to boost your nutritional levels. I focus on teas in this chapter and talk about infusions much more in Chapter 10.

One of the best things about teas is that they're so easy to make. They only require two ingredients, herbs and water. Teas also come in two main variations, hot and cold. Each has its advantages. Hot teas are quicker to make, and they're better at extracting minerals and resinous compounds from the herb. They can also extract a much higher amount of essential oils from the plant. Cold teas take longer to make, although no more effort, and are better at extracting polysaccharides and bitter components. Although they are a bit less efficient at pulling out essential oil, cold teas do a much better job protecting the potent ingredients in the oil than hot teas are able to do. For this reason, plants with very active essential oils are often prepared cold.

However, you're not committing any great herbal sin if you use a tea preparation that is not thought to be preferred for a particular herb. Through exploration, you will discover how to personalize your brews and draw out an herb's maximum power.

Teas (and infusions) are wonderfully simple, but they come with a couple of small downsides. First of all, once brewed, they have a short shelf life. A tea will stay potent for 1 day without refrigeration and for about 2 to 3 days with refrigeration. You can't make a big batch to last you all week. Another limitation is that, although water is good at extracting many things, it can't extract everything. If you have a plant that's sticky, oily, waxy, or resinous, water likely will not be your best extractor. Thankfully, you have other methods to help prepare these plants, which you'll learn about very soon.

Making Teas

Of course, everyone knows how to make tea, but please don't skip over this section because there's an important additional step you need to take when you are making teas for medicine.

To make a hot tea, place your herbs in a cup and pour boiling water over them. For most applications, you can use 1 cup of water with about 1 to 3 teaspoons of dried herbs or 1 to 2 tablespoons of fresh herbs.

Then, immediately place a saucer or other lid over the cup. This important step holds in heat and traps any essential oils or other volatile medicinal compounds inside the cup. If you don't get that lid on quickly, these valuable components quickly evaporate and escape.

When the tea has cooled enough to drink, tip up the saucer, letting any condensation fall back into your tea. Add honey or lemon, if desired, and drink up.

For cold teas, place your herbs in a cup and pour clean, room temperature water over them. Again, you can use 1 cup of water with 1 to 3 teaspoons of dried herbs or 1 to 2 tablespoons of fresh herbs. Place a cover over your tea, this time to prevent dust or bugs from getting in it, and let the tea sit overnight, or for at least 8 hours, at room temperature before drinking.

With either method, you can place your herbs in a teabag, a tea ball, or any similar device. You could also let the herbs dance freely in the water as they infuse and strain them out before you drink. Or don't strain them at all. Those herb remnants will still have a little medicine in them, so if the texture doesn't bother you, just drink them with the liquid.

For most herbs and conditions, 3 or 4 cups of tea a day is a nice amount.

Tea Tips

- If you make more tea than you can drink, freeze it in ice cube trays. When you're ready for it, place a few cubes in a glass and sip them throughout the day as they melt.

- If you're in a hurry, you can jump-start a cold tea by pulsing it in a blender for several seconds.

- Did your mother or grandmother ever make sun tea? That is a variation of the cold method. Simply place your tea in direct sunlight. As the tea infuses, it will also become charged with solar energy that gently warms and circulates the liquid.

- Moon tea is another cold tea variation. Make it the same as sun tea, but at night. Be sure to place it where the moonlight will shine into your container.

- For either sun or moon tea, use a clear container to let the light in.

healing with teas

Peppermint tea is wonderful to help calm an upset stomach. If you've got a youngster prone to carsickness, once you get to where you're going, make a mug of peppermint tea with a touch of honey to help calm that little belly. The mint leaves have anti-inflammatory properties that help soothe muscles in the stomach and intestines. I've found peppermint tea is also great to help clear my mind, especially when business meetings go on and on.

Ginger is one of my favorite go-to teas for immune support. The first time I had ginger tea, I was living in Hong Kong and came down with a bad chest infection. My Filipino housekeeper chopped some fresh ginger into approximately ¼ cup of pea-sized pieces and simmered them on the stove in a quart of water for about 10 minutes. Then she strained out the bulk and insisted I drink the spicy concoction every few hours. It helped tremendously, and I've loved ginger tea ever since. In the winter, I drink ginger tea to naturally warm my body from the inside. Like peppermint, ginger is an anti-inflammatory and good for any kind of stomach upset.

Lemon balm, also known as Melissa, has a citrusy taste, as you would guess from the name. This tea uplifts your mood and helps clear your mind. It is reputed to help improve memory, and it contains high concentrations of antioxidants that detoxify the body.

Guayusa is a caffeinated tea with a kick similar to coffee, but without the jitters. I've come to love the gentler form of caffeine and the earthy taste of guayusa tea. Guayusa is not well known in the United States, although it has been used for centuries by indigenous people in the rainforests. Early medical studies on guayusa report high levels of antioxidants and immune-supporting factors.

Don't limit yourself to single-herb teas. Mixing and matching and creating delicious blends is also very fun.

Tea Rituals

There's one last secret power of tea: *ritual*. The Japanese have made tea drinking an art form, but you don't need to have that kind of elaborate ceremony to achieve a lot of the same results. Just creating a small ritual of your own can help bring more harmony and tranquility into your life.

Tea rituals help establish rhythms and attach meaning to our actions. Each night, as I get ready for bed, I like to make a cup of chamomile tea and prepare an infusion for the next morning. (See Chapter 10 for more information on preparing infusions.) Instead of just mindlessly putting the water on to boil, I like to spend that time being as present in the moment as I can. I am very aware of my hands turning on the water and filling the teapot. I notice my breath. I feel my body movements as I turn to place the pot on the stove. I smell the herbs and appreciate them as I prepare the jars I like to drink from. For a brief second I try to see the sunlight captured in the dried flowers of the chamomile and sense the rain that fell on them while they were growing. Then, I head off to brush my teeth, and by the time I'm finished, the teakettle is just starting to sing. It's a cycle that repeats night after night, amplifying my natural body rhythms and signaling my mind and body to start winding down for sleep.

You can create your own tea rituals for waking up, going to bed, destressing after work, regularly connecting with a friend, or any other occasion. When you start to get sick, you'll likely find that the sounds and smells of tea-making help you feel better even before you drink the tea.

Tinctures, Vinegars, and Glycerites

A tincture is a liquid extract using alcohol. (I talk about its cousins, glycerites and vinegars, in a moment.) Tinctures have several great qualities. They're portable, easy to make, and have a very long shelf life. A properly stored tincture will last many years or even decades, so you can make a lot in advance to prepare for an emergency. They're also very concentrated, meaning you can get a lot of effect with smaller doses. Tinctures are also great for when you're working with bark, roots, or other tough materials that might be difficult to process. You can also use them to preserve rare herbs.

One time I was at a gathering where a fellow was selling stills to make your own alcohol. I couldn't help but tease my friends Cat and Hal Farneman as they circled the still, asking questions while obviously looking to buy. Cat and Hal are devout Mormons, and if you didn't know, their faith prohibits the consumption of alcohol. In retrospect, I am a little embarrassed at my teasing them because Cat created the herbal medicine company Purr-fectly Herbal by Cat. She and Hal took my ribbing with good nature and gently explained to me that their small community had pooled together the money for her to buy a still so she could have alcohol to make tinctures. Mormons have a strong ethic of preparedness, and being able to make and store medicines is vitally important to them.

Making Tinctures

There are many ways to make a tincture, but we're going to look at the simplest and most traditional method.

Start by chopping your fresh herbs into small chunks, perhaps the size of corn kernels. The finer you chop the herbs, roots, or bark, the better the extraction, but you don't need to go overboard. Put your chopped herbs in a jar, and fill the jar with vodka or another strong alcohol. I like to use organic vodka, but this is really up to you. Keep pouring until the herbs are covered by about ½ inch of alcohol. Add the lid.

Next, label your jar. Write down the name of herb(s) used, the kind and strength of the alcohol, and the date it was started. You'll never regret good record-keeping. I can't tell you how many jars of unlabeled stuff I have that I really wish I had taken the time to label. Note that it is best to label the jar itself and not the lid because lids have a habit of traveling around and just can't be trusted.

Be sure the lid is tight, and shake the jar well. Place it in a cupboard or some other place out of sunlight. Come back and shake the jar every few days or once a week. Remember to speak encouraging words to it, as you would with a glycerite or vinegar. Tinctures are generally considered done after a month, although you can let them go longer without harm.

When you have finished the extraction process, strain out the plant material by pouring the jar's contents through a fine mesh strainer, piece of muslin, or other cloth set over a bowl. Be sure to squeeze out all the liquid you can. Rebottle the liquid, and your tincture is ready to use! (Be sure to compost those spent herbs, too.)

The strength of your alcohol is important. A vodka of 80 to 100 proof (40 to 50 percent alcohol) is suitable for most dry herbs. If you're using fresh herbs, you'll want to use a much stronger alcohol of perhaps 180 or 190 proof (90 to 95 percent alcohol). The fresh herbs already have a lot of water in them, so you need more alcohol or the mixture will have a tendency to mold or rot instead of preserve. Alcohol of this strength will have enough power to extract medicinal compounds and prevent bacterial growth. It will also have a favorable ratio of alcohol to water, pulling out the maximum variety of medicinal components. The alcohol can pull out what the water can't, and the water can pull out what the alcohol can't. They make a great team.

Essential oils, berries, and succulent herbs extract better with stronger-proof alcohol, up to 140 proof (70 percent alcohol). For gums and resins, use 180 proof (90 percent alcohol).

Tincture Tips

- Use only ethanol alcohol. That's the kind of alcohol found in wine, beer, and other alcoholic drinks. Rubbing alcohol is not an acceptable substitute. It is highly toxic when taken internally.

- It won't hurt a thing to leave the herbs in the jar longer than the time specified. Some people leave them for months until they finally get ready to use the tincture.

- You can jump-start the extraction process by pulsing the herbs and alcohol in a blender a few times.

- Store tinctures in dark, well-labeled bottles out of the light.

Making Herbal Vinegars

An herbal vinegar is made just like a tincture, except you use vinegar instead of alcohol. I make my herbal vinegars with a good-quality apple cider vinegar that is "alive," such as Bragg Organic Apple Cider Vinegar.

Herbal vinegars are often used in cooking, and the herbs typically used in the vinegars reflect this. Rosemary (*Rosmarinus officinalis*), thyme (*Thymus vulgaris*), garlic (*Allium sativum*), sage (*Salvia officinalis*), lavender (*Lavandula* sp.), and elderberries (*Sambucus nigra*) are all great choices. These herbs create delicious vinegars that give dishes a kick of flavor and punch up the health value.

Some herbal vinegars are specifically made to increase your nutritional levels. Nettles (*Urtica dioica*), alfalfa (*Medicago sativa*), dandelion (*Taraxacum officinale*), and cleavers (*Galium aparine*) are rich in calcium, phosphorus, potassium, iron, and more, and the vinegar is excellent at extracting these minerals and making them more available to you. When you are making herbal vinegars for the nutritional boost, be sure to use a lot of plant material—as much as you can stuff in that jar—before covering with the vinegar.

You can make vinegars with other herbs for specific medicinal qualities, too, if you just don't want to consume the alcohol used in tinctures.

Vinegars don't last nearly as long as alcohol tinctures, and how long they last seems to be a topic of debate. My nettles vinegar was fine for over a year, and it might have gone longer, but I used it all.

Making Glycerites

The last variation is a glycerite. Glycerites are made with vegetable glycerin and have the advantage of tasting sweet. Even the most reluctant kids (and spouses) will take them. Glycerites are also a good option for people who want to avoid alcohol. Glycerites do require refrigeration and have a shorter shelf life of 6 months to a year. Glycerin is also a weaker extractor than alcohol. It works better with leaves and flowers than roots and bark. Just be sure to use coarse herbs when making a glycerite. Powdered herbs can make straining very difficult.

The process for making glycerites is similar to making tincture, but you substitute vegetable glycerin for the alcohol.

Dilute the glycerin with distilled water, using two parts water to three parts glycerin.

Next, just as you would with an alcohol tincture, fill a jar with your dried herbs until it's mostly full. Then, fill the jar completely with your glycerin-water mixture, making sure you've got about ½ inch of liquid covering the herbs on top. Add the lid.

Place the mixture in your refrigerator to begin the extraction process. Glycerin doesn't have the same preservation power as alcohol and can't be left out on the counter. Remember to shake it and speak encouraging words to it, as you would with a tincture or vinegar. After a few weeks, filter out the herbs and place the mixture back in the fridge.

Dosage

How much of these tinctures, vinegars, or glycerites should you use? First, let me put your mind at ease by saying that most common herbs are actually very safe. In fact, they're much safer than prescription or over-the-counter medications. You'd have to try *really* hard to overdo it with chamomile (*Matricaria chamomilla, Chamaemelum nobile*), nettles (*Urtica dioica*), or echinacea (*Echinacea purpurea*).

There are a few herbs you should be more cautious with, like lobelia (*Lobelia inflata, L. cardinalis*), and you should always go slow the first time you try any new herb to see how your body will react. But in general, you've got a lot of wiggle room with herbal medicine.

Herbal vinegars created specifically for their medicinal value can be dosed similarly to tinctures and glycerites. But if you are using your herbal vinegars for culinary or nutritional purposes, you don't have to think in terms of "dosages," but rather how well they taste or fit in a recipe. Typically, you'll use much larger quantities of culinary and nutritive vinegars because they are made with culinary herbs or herbals foods. Use them freely. You'll get sick of the taste long before you get sick from the herb.

Tinctures and glycerite dosages are typically dispensed by a dropper and, therefore, are measured in either drops or dropperfuls. A typical adult dose for a tincture or glycerite is 1 dropperful. This is, admittedly, imprecise, and again, really all herbal medicine is very imprecise. For example, it's hard to know how strong the medicine is in the roots you've harvested. If you harvested in the late autumn, the potency of your roots is stronger than in roots harvested midsummer. There are a lot of variables, but one of the great things about herbal medicine is that there is so much room for personalization. You can fine-tune remedies and dosages to fit your and your family's needs exactly.

You may find that your body responds well to a certain herb and you may not need as large a dose as someone else. Your body can also crave more of a certain herb than another. Listen to your body. Let it, and the plants, guide you. You'll always have more success by working in a fluid way, rather than working from a static formula. Just go slowly, and keep checking in with your body.

Liniments

Liniments are basically tinctures used externally. You can use any tincture as a liniment, but you should never use a liniment as a tincture. Liniments are often made with rubbing alcohol and/or herbs that should not be taken internally. Rubbing alcohol is a much less expensive option and is safe to use on the skin, but it is highly toxic when ingested.

Make a liniment precisely as you would make a tincture. Feel free to swap the relatively more expensive vodka with rubbing alcohol. When you are finished, be sure to clearly mark your container "external use only."

Apply a liniment by pouring it over the desired area and rubbing it in by hand. If that isn't convenient, you can try the following strategies:

- Use a spray bottle.

- Soak a cloth and lay it over the affected area.

- Mix it with olive oil and rub it onto the skin.

healing with liniments

Liniments used to be a lot more common in household medicine chests because, historically, lifestyles were more active.

My favorite way to use liniments is for soothing sore muscles and achy joints. Arnica (*Arnica montana*) is a flower that has a real affinity for helping muscles and joints. It's my standard go-to if I wake up stiff from too much physical activity the day before. Sometimes I'll add rosemary to my arnica liniment to stimulate circulation. This helps speed healing and clear lactic acid from my overused muscles. If I apply it before going to bed, I can decrease, and even often prevent, next-day soreness. It's also great for bruises and sprains. Arnica and peppermint is another really lovely combination. It's very cold at first, but then it heats up and feels great—a bit like an herbal IcyHot.

amazing adaptogenic herbs

Adaptogens are the superstars of the herbal world. They help boost energy, restore vitality, and improve the body's ability to deal with the stresses of modern-day life. The elders in our herbal community, and a growing body of scientific research, teach that these are the best herbs for increasing life force and promoting longevity.

An herb can be classified as an adaptogen if it meets these three criteria:

1. It is nontoxic and safe to use over a long period of time. It can be taken daily for years, and your body will continue to love it.

2. It is a true generalist and doesn't have a specific action in the body. In other words, it's not used for one specific condition or organ system, but rather to tonify and support your entire system.

3. It has a normalizing effect in the body, which means it often simply does what the body needs to restore balance and health.

The term "adaptogen" is fairly new, and you won't find it in any of the herb books printed before 1985. But these herbs have been around for generations. They come from Chinese, Indian-Vedic, and global indigenous traditions.

Traditionally, these herbs were simply incorporated into meals, and that is the preferred way most of our herbal community elders use them. They put them in soups and stews, sneak them into batches of cookies, or simply sprinkle the powdered herbs into food. You can make them into syrups, herbal teas, or delicious spreads, too. Some of these herbs are not that pleasant tasting, so taking them as homemade pills or tinctures gets them down easier. I like to mix several of these herbs (about 1 teaspoon of each powdered herb) and put them in an oat milk smoothie at the end of the day. Feel free to experiment with what feels right to you.

Probably the biggest benefit of regularly taking adaptogens is how much they help with stress relief. I find it fascinating that most of these adaptogens are weedy species that grow in very harsh, stressful environments, yet they grow with stunning beauty and poise. Because these plants are masters of living well in difficult environments, it makes sense they can help with our stressful situations.

Following is a list and brief description of some of the best adaptogens, all of which increase your overall ability to adapt and to resist stress. Remember, as with all the herbs mentioned in this book, please try these in small test quantities in the rare case your body doesn't like the herb.

Also note that these adaptogenic herbs don't work quickly. They need to be used over a period of time, usually at least a month, before you notice anything. They are also very gentle. Because they're so beneficial for restoring life force and body energy, it's good to incorporate these into your lifestyle as food.

Ginseng. American ginseng (*Panax quinquefolius*) and related species are probably the world's best-known adaptogens. Ginseng is an herb that helps restore energy and aids the chronically ill. It also helps build overall stamina and strength. It is so well known and useful, it has been far overharvested and is severely at risk in its native habitat. For this reason, I absolutely don't recommend using it.

The great news is, another option is available that is much more abundant, easier to grow, more cost effective, and yet has the same amazing properties. Siberian ginseng (*Eleutherococcus senticosus*) is not a true ginseng, but it is a close relative that contains almost the exact same properties. It has an impressive range of health benefits and thousands of studies have been done by Russian scientists proving its ability to increase endurance and stamina. Russian athletes measured a 9 percent improvement in stamina when taking Siberian ginseng for only a month, and 1,000 factory workers who took three dropperfuls of Siberian ginseng extract daily showed a 40 percent reduction in the number of sick days taken.

Unlike American ginseng, Siberian ginseng is found growing in abundance over a large range, and it is much more cost effective and ecologically viable. As you can guess from its name, the plant really loves cold, harsh climates. It can be grown in the northern part of the United States and into Canada. The root is the medicine.

Burdock (*Arctium lappa*) is that weed with the big leaves you've probably seen growing in fields and along the roadsides. It is most famous for its big, spiky sticker balls that contain the seeds of the plant. Those spiky balls were the inspiration for the design of Velcro. A friend of mine says that if you get burdock stickers on your socks, forget getting them out and just start watering the socks, and you'll grow a nice little patch of burdock.

The whole burdock plant is useful, but the root is the wonderful adaptogenic herb that's very restorative to the body. It's deeply nourishing, with a rich concentration of vitamin B_6, manganese, potassium, phosphorus, folate, calcium, and iron. Burdock has a special affinity for the liver, and it helps with liver congestion and sluggish liver.

It's also really good for skin issues. Many herbalists use it with teenagers and young adults because over a period of time, it's very restorative to the skin and complexion.

If you are new to herbalism, you might be scratching your head and wondering how these herbs can do so many apparently very different things. How can burdock help with both the liver and the skin? As you learn more about your body's systems, organs, and chemistry, you'll see that, yes, it all does make sense. In this case, because you are exposed to so many pollutants every day, your liver has to filter and clean your blood of those pollutants. If your liver is overwhelmed, the pollutants will continue on through the blood and be pushed out through the skin. So if you help your liver, your skin problems will clear up, too.

Burdock roots are also a very tasty food. In Japan, it's called gobo root and is a highly prized addition to meals. You can flavor it and cook it just like carrots. The roots are best harvested in the autumn of the plant's first year, before the plant goes to seed in the following year. It's a great plant to wild-craft because it's a very weedy species and you won't hurt it by taking some.

Ashwagandha (*Withania somnifera*) is a plant that comes from the ancient ayurvedic system of healing. The dried and powdered root of the plant is the medicine. It's generally grown as a perennial, and although it likes to grow in a hot, sunny area, even in northern climates you can get a big root out of a single growing season. Ashwagandha, sometimes referred to as "Indian ginseng" although it is not a ginseng at all, is highly regarded as an herb that increases memory, facilitates learning, and in general makes you relax all over (although it's also considered a sexual tonic).

Ashwagandha has a kind of peculiar taste and odor. Although it's not really bad tasting, it's not necessarily good tasting either. That's why it's often blended with more flavorful herbs such as ginger, chai, cinnamon, or sarsaparilla. In India, where it is probably the most popular herb to drink in the evening, it's mixed with warm milk, honey, and cinnamon to improve the flavor.

Ashwagandha belongs to the Solanaceae family, the same family as potatoes, eggplant, and tomatoes. The aerial part of almost all those plants is toxic, so don't eat the berries or the leaves. The root is the medicine.

Astragalus (*Astragalus membranaceus*) is one of the most outstanding herbs for building deep immune strength, and it helps rebuild bone marrow reserves, which is where your immune cells are born. Herbalists speak of astragalus's ability to support and regenerate the body's "protective shield." I know that doesn't really make sense in medical terminology, but it makes sense in herbalism, which has a more holistic approach. As an immune system builder, astragalus is used both to prevent and treat long-term infections, including chronic colds, repeating flus, and candida. One study published by the American Cancer Society reported that a water extract of astragalus improved immune function in 90 percent of cancer patients studied. And in studies done over an 8-year period by the National Cancer Research Institution and five other research institutes, astragalus was shown to improve the immune system of cancer patients as well as lessen the negative side effects of the cancer treatment.

Astragalus is an easy herb to grow. It's a legume, Fabaceae, in the pea family. The root is the medicine.

Schisandra berries (*Schisandra chinensis*) are called the "five-flavored plant" in Chinese medicine because they have five distinctive flavors: sweet, salty, sour, pungent, and bitter. As you're chewing the little berries, you get each flavor in sequence until you have the entire taste sensation—it's really an amazing experience. In traditional Chinese medicine, each flavor attaches to a specific organ system. Schisandra berries are considered a superior medicine because they have all five flavors, which activate and balance all the different organs.

Classified as an adaptogen herb for raising the body's ability to resist all manner of stress and disease, schisandra berries were used primarily by wealthy, upper-middle-class Chinese women as a preserver of youth, a beauty aid, and a powerful female sexual tonic. This is one of the few herbs classified as a *female* sexual tonic. Generally, sexual tonics can be used equally by both men and women, but traditionally they are mostly for men.

Researchers found that racehorses on schisandra berries not only increased their 800-meter time from 52.2 to 50.4 seconds—a competitive advantage of six lengths—but their breathing and heart rates returned to normal faster than those horses given the placebo.

The plant is also called magnolia vine, and you can buy it at nurseries. The medicine is the bluish berries. I like the berries, but try them for yourself because they do have a distinct flavor. I sometimes like to take a small bag of dried berries on a hike with me for a snack. They are great in teas and syrups, added to jams and jellies, and almost any way you would eat other berries.

Holy basil (*Ocimum tenuiflorum*), whose common name is tulsi, which means "the unmatched" or "the incomparable one," is, like all the adaptogens, helpful for reducing stress, increasing energy and vitality, and promoting longevity. Holy basil is widely used in India today and is certainly one of the most highly regarded herbs, with more than 3,000 years of recorded medicinal use in ayurvedic medicine. The daily use of this herb is believed to help maintain the balance of the chakras and bring out the goodness, virtue, and joy in humans.

Holy basil is a very pleasant-tasting herb that I find nice just by itself in tea. And it's also fun to mix with rose hips, peppermint, lemon balm, and whatever else you've got to experiment with.

Holy basil can be used much like sweet basil, although the flavors are definitely different, and you can use it to season food just like any of the basils. If you make a holy basil pesto, start with a small amount. Maybe mix it with sweet basil and other culinary herbs because the flavor will be different. Most people enjoy the taste.

Just like the other basils, holy basil is an easy-to-grow annual that grows rapidly. You harvest the leaves regularly to use fresh or to dry for later. It's nice to plant in a pot by your front door.

Gotu kola (*Centella asiatica*) also has a long history of use, and like the other adaptogens, helps with so many aspects of improving health. Gotu kola is most famous for improving memory and clearing the mind. In small mountain villages in India, groups of people commonly live to be in their 90s and 100s, with no dementia whatsoever. In fact, they are renowned for their remarkable mental acuity. The people of these villages credit the gotu kola, which they don't use as a medicinal plant, but as a daily green.

In areas of Thailand where gotu kola grows, people eat a few leaves as an afternoon pick-me-up because it increases and restores energy. I've heard that elephants in the wild choose gotu kola as a favorite food—and we all know elephants are renowned for their remarkable memories!

Gotu kola is a beautiful little ground cover that grows wild in many tropical regions of the world. Everywhere it's grown, it's considered a remarkable food and herb. You can also grow it in pots and bring it indoors when it gets cold. You only need a few of the little green leaves every day. They do have a bitter taste, but you are not eating a lot.

Milky oats (*Avena sativa*) are among the best tonic herbs for the nervous system and are also a superior cardiovascular tonic. If you find yourself overworked, stressed, and anxious, consider including milky oats in your daily health program. The milky oat tops are rich in silica, calcium, chromium, and magnesium, which help explain in part their medicinal properties and their beneficial effect on the nervous system. They are also rich in vitamin E and polyunsaturated fatty acids, which are important for vitality.

Some herbalists report milky oats are also really good for sexual vitality, citing that a tincture of milky oats can increase friskiness.

The reason they are called milky oats is because you harvest the newly forming oat seeds before they mature. If you squeeze the seed case, a droplet of a milky substance comes out. The seeds are in this stage only for about a week per season, so you have to catch them at the right time. Don't worry if you miss it because the fully ripe oats are simply oatmeal and that is also extremely nutritious, full of fiber, and good for heart health. But for making medicine, herbalists really like oats harvested in the milky stage.

Infused Oils, Salves, and Lotions

One of the things I love about airports is seeing the open expressions of love between people who are either departing from each other or coming back from a faraway journey. This is one of the places in America where we openly and tenderly hug and touch one another.

Touch is such a powerful healing force. Part of the healing magic in this section of preparations is based on touch. Most moms know that a child screaming from a fresh boo-boo will almost immediately forget about it after the wound has been cleaned, a healing salve gently applied, and the bandage set. A large part of the healing has to do with the attention and gentle touch Mom gives the wound (and, therefore, the child).

Infused oils, salves, and lotions are all about soothing. They don't evaporate quickly, making them a longer-lasting option for the skin than a liniment. Plus, they draw on the power of a loving hand, which connects us to one another more meaningfully and intimately than a cup of tea or a dropper of tincture. In a time when our society is separated by technology and often even afraid to reach out to one another, meaningful physical contact is absolutely vital to our physical and emotional wellness. And for those of you who are interested in making your own cosmetics, infused oils, salves, and lotions are a great entry into that world.

Infused oils, salves, and lotions are best made in smaller batches and stored in your refrigerator because they don't have long shelf lives. Depending on the oils and other ingredients you use, expect only about 1 to 6 months.

Making Infused Oils

To make a salve or lotion, you need an infused oil as a base. So let's start there. Infusing an oil is easy and can be done in two ways.

The first method is faster, and it's the way I usually make my oils. Place your herbs and oil in a double boiler over medium heat. (And you really do want to use a double boiler. If you heat the oil directly on the stovetop, you risk cooking out the medicinal properties.) Let the oil and herbs infuse for 30 minutes to 1 hour. When it's ready, the oil will have absorbed the color and smell of the herbs, and the herbs will look dead and spent. Strain out the herbs, rebottle the oil, and refrigerate it. Refrigeration isn't strictly necessary, but it will extend the usable life of your oil. Good oil should smell clean or have the scent of the infused herbs. If it smells rancid, it's time to compost it.

The second method is slower, but it's better at protecting the herb's medicinal components, and it's an off-grid solution that uses a natural energy source—the sun. Place the dried herbs in a jar, and cover them with a natural oil, such as olive, almond, jojoba, or coconut. Seal the jar, place it in a brown paper bag, and set it on a warm (not hot) windowsill for 1 to 2 weeks. Then strain and rebottle as instructed in the double-boiler method.

To use an infused oil, just rub it right on your skin as often as needed. I know what some of you are thinking: *Wouldn't that be awfully . . . oily?* Yes, it is very oily, and many people don't like that sensation on their skin. The solution? Turn that infused oil into a salve or lotion!

Infused Oil Tip

• If you make an infused oil with coconut oil, use either the hot method or use the slower method in the summer. Coconut oil will solidify on cool days, greatly reducing its ability to extract medicines from the herbs.

Making Salves

A salve is just an oil that's been thickened with beeswax. Salves are considerably less messy than oils and work great as lip balms.

To make a salve, warm your infused oil in a double boiler over medium heat. Add 1 ounce of beeswax (by weight) for every 1 cup of oil. Stir until the beeswax has melted completely, pour the mixture into a jar or lip balm–style container, and let it cool.

Salve Tip

• Use a wide-mouth jar when storing your salves. This makes it much easier to reach in and get out what you need.

Making Lotions

One of the things I enjoy about the women who live in deserts is that many of them make their own lotions. The climate there is so dry, but these women have figured out ways to keep their skin looking young and moist even in extreme conditions. Your face is especially sensitive skin, so it is well worth making your own lotions to be certain of the purity of the ingredients. (The beauty industry is notorious for using all kinds of stabilizers and preservatives, which are essentially toxic). Another bonus: lotions are easy to make.

A lotion is the next step beyond a salve. It's softer and easier to apply. Plus, you can be creative if you like, by adding in all kinds of extra herbs, essential oils, or even tinctures.

To make a lotion, warm your salve back up in the double boiler over medium heat. Or continue from there if you've just made your salve. Add 1 cup of water for every 1 cup of oil you have. Or for more potency, replace the water with an herbal infusion.

When everything is melted, remove the double boiler from the heat, and use an immersion blender to carefully whip the mixture until your lotion has increased in volume and become luxuriantly smooth. (A regular blender works, too, but it's much harder to get clean.)

Lotion Tip

- When you're blending a lotion, feel free to add essential oils and tinctures. Experimenting is fun!

healing with infused oils, salves, and lotions

Relieve minor sprains. One of my favorite herbs to use to make infused oil is turmeric (*Curcuma longa*). I use about ¼ cup of finely chopped turmeric with about 1 cup of coconut oil. The oil turns bright orange as it takes on the potent anti-inflammatory properties of turmeric. I've used this oil for several injuries, including a nagging sprain or something wrong in my ankle that refused to heal. After I started applying the turmeric oil, my ankle finally relaxed and got over the injury.

Hydrate your lips. I don't recommend using turmeric as a lip balm unless you want bright yellow lips! But making a lip balm with licorice or a little cherry extract can give your lip salve a pleasing flavor. Kids love this project.

Nourish your skin. Lotions made with calendula flowers (*Calendula officinalis*), chamomile (*Matricaria recutita, Chamaemelum nobile*), and comfrey (*Symphytum officinale*) are known to be soothing to the skin.

Homemade antibiotic ointment. Make a homemade Neosporin equivalent for those little scrapes, cuts, and bites. For the salve, blend calendula flowers (*Calendula officinalis*), which are so soothing to the skin; comfrey (*Symphytum officinale*), which is an awesome healer; and lavender (*Lavandula angustifolia*), which is an amazing antibiotic. Get the kids involved in making the salve. They'll remember they helped, which will give the salve extra potency for their injuries.

Syrups and Gelatins

No matter how effective an herbal remedy is, it's not going to do anyone any good if you can't get them to take it. Children (and spouses) can be quite picky about what they eat or drink. Thankfully, there's a sweet solution. Delicious herbal syrups and gelatins will be favorites with everyone, even the fussiest family members.

Making Elderberry Syrup (Basic Syrup Recipe)

Elderberry syrup is the most famous herbal syrup preparation, and I always have some on hand. Its antimicrobial and immune-boosting properties have gotten me and my family through many cold and flu seasons over the years.

To make a syrup, you first need elderberry juice. Place ¼ cup of dried elderberries (*Sambucus nigra*) and 1 cup of water in a pan on the stove over medium heat, and let it simmer for 20 minutes.

While it's simmering, you might want to toss in some cloves (*Syzygium aromaticum*), cinnamon (*Cinnamomum* sp.), ginger (*Zingiber officinale*), or cardamom (*Elettaria cardamomum*). These spices give your syrup an exotic, warming flavor, and they also pack additional immune-supporting power.

Let the juice cool (even overnight is fine) and then strain it. A clean cloth handkerchief works well for straining. Give it a good squeeze to get out all the precious liquid. Compost the leftover berry mush, or give it to your chickens.

You'll probably have around ½ cup of liquid at this point. Add ½ cup of honey and mix well.

Congratulations! You just made elderberry syrup.

Can you use another sweetener besides honey? Yes, but the less processed your sweetener is, the better. Raw honey is always the healthiest choice. It has antimicrobial and other healing properties that are passed along to you in the syrup.

Note: If you are using honey and it isn't dissolving, you can heat it gently. Don't heat it too much because you don't want to harm the honey's medicinal properties. When your honey and elderberry juice are well combined, pour the syrup into a clean glass container and add a lid. Be sure to label the jar with all the ingredients and the date it was created. Your syrup will last at least 2 weeks in the refrigerator, if you don't eat it all before then.

How do you use elderberry syrup? Just take 1 or 2 tablespoons like you would any cough syrup. But unlike other cough syrups, you can pour elderberry syrup on pancakes, oatmeal, yogurt, muffins, or fruit. Yum! You can even add a spoonful or two to carbonated water to make your own herbal soda.

Syrup Tip

- You can go beyond the elderberry and make all kinds of syrups that still have great health benefits. Use the same recipe as for elderberry syrup, and just replace the berries with your choice of herbs or other ingredients. Schisandra berries (*Schisandra chinensis*) are a wonderful adaptogen, generally beneficial and toning to the whole body. Ginger, cloves, and cinnamon make a delightfully warming syrup with lots of immune-boosting qualities, too. Feel free to experiment and mix and match ingredients.

Making Gelatins

For another fun option, you can transform your syrup into an herbal gelatin. This is definitely a great way to get herbs into your family's diet. To make herbal gelatin, you'll need the following ingredients:

> 1 cup syrup (Elderberry is terrific!)
>
> 2 tablespoons unflavored gelatin powder
>
> ½ cup hot (not boiling) water or juice
>
> A bit of oil (Coconut is great, or any oil without a strong taste.)

Pour ¼ cup of herbal syrup into a 2-cup measuring cup. (If you just made the syrup, let it cool first.) Whisk in the gelatin.

Add the hot water or juice, and whisk until smooth. Instead of plain water, you can substitute an herbal infusion, which will give the gelatin an extra punch of herbal goodness. Add the rest of the syrup, and whisk until everything is smooth.

Lightly oil an 8×8-inch pan. Pour the gelatin mixture into the prepared pan, and refrigerate for about 2 hours or until the gelatin is set.

Poultices

Poultices are a topical application, great for rashes, burns, bites, stings, cuts, and other surface-level injuries. Poultices are one of the critical methods of dealing with infected wounds, and they really are very effective. Their benefits also go deeper (literally). The skin easily absorbs many plant compounds. This means a poultice can be placed over deep bruises, sprained ligaments, internal organs, or even broken bones to deliver healing where it is needed.

Herbs used in poultices are usually chosen for their ability to heal wounds, kill bacteria, soothe pain and inflammation, and draw out infection or foreign materials. Plantain (*Plantago* sp.), comfrey (*Symphytum officinale*), calendula (*Calendula officinalis*), chickweed (*Sellaria media*), marshmallow root (*Althaea officinalis*), chamomile (*Matricaria recutita, Chamaemelum nobile*), and prickly pear (*Opuntia* sp.) innards are all great choices for poultices. Even common cabbage makes a great poultice, as I mentioned earlier.

There are two basic rules with poultices: make a larger amount of poultice than you think you need, and keep it on the area you are trying to heal for longer than you think you need to do so.

Making and Applying Poultices

To make a poultice, simply mix the herbs with water to form a wet mash. If the herb, such as cabbage or prickly pear, is already moist, you don't need to add much water. To make a poultice with prickly pear pads, you'll first need to take care of the needles. The fastest and easiest way to do this is to rub two rocks all over the pad surface while the pad is still attached to the plant. This way, the plant holds the pad for you. Don't forget the edges. Then you can snap off the pad, chop it up, and run it through the blender to make a nice slurry.

Apply the poultice very thickly in an area at least twice as large as the affected spot—four to ten times larger is better. So if you have a wound about the size of a quarter (about 1 inch in diameter), have your poultice cover the wound and surrounding area in the size of a softball (about 4 inches in diameter). Use a towel or wrap to hold the poultice in place. I'm not a big user of plastic wrap, but this is a situation it is really good for. Leave the poultice in place for several hours. Overnight is great.

When you remove the poultice and clean and gently pat dry the wound and surrounding area, you should see some progress, if not complete healing. Apply a fresh poultice if needed, leaving it on as long as you did the first one. If you aren't seeing good progress within a few days, it might be time to seek help from a trusted health-care provider.

The two main mistakes people make with poultices are that they don't use enough plant material and they don't leave it on long enough. Remember, you need enough poultice material to cover the wound and a large part of the surrounding area. It's not enough to just cover the sore alone; you've got to cover the surrounding area, too. Poultices work with amazing results, but you've got to have some patience. This is not a 10-minute process. Remember, go big, and go for a long time!

the next generation

An herbalist friend of mine, Scott Sexton, knows the importance of passing on our herbal medicine knowledge to the next generation. One day, his 3-year-old daughter, Katy, was out playing under some fruit trees when she was stung by a fire ant. Her 4-year-old brother, Lincoln, proudly declared, "I know what to do," and ran into a nearby field. He returned with a handful of plantain leaves, which he chewed up and applied to Katy's bite.

With the pain gone, Katy thanked her brother with a hug, and the two went back to playing. Lincoln hadn't just learned about a plant. He'd also learned that he could protect and take care of his younger sister.

When it comes to herbal medicines, you can never start teaching them too soon.

Poultice Tips

- Supercharge a poultice by mixing the herbs with an infusion rather than water. You could add a tincture, too. Medicine-makers are always getting creative to find new and better solutions.

- Although dry herbs are more common, fresh herbs can be used in poultices. Just be sure they are crushed or blended enough to release their medicines.

- The simplest form of poultice is called a "spit poultice." This is when you chew an herb in your mouth and apply it to the skin. It's often done with plantain leaves because that is a super-common plant everywhere. It may sound gross, but if you ever get stung when you're far out in the woods, you'll be glad you know about it.

- You can make poultices ahead of time and freeze them until they're needed. Just spread them out on a square of cheesecloth, slide them into individual zipper-close bags, and place them in your freezer.

There are many other ways to prepare plants in herbal preparations, but once you've got these eight down, you are well on your way to becoming a medicine woman or man. When you reach this stage, you may not hear any blaring trumpets, nor will you get a big blue ribbon. But perhaps one day you'll have a new friend over and she will open your kitchen cabinet and see the jars of dried herbs, the dropper bottles of tinctures, and the homemade herbal vinegars on your counter, all with neatly hand-written labels. She will turn to you with one eyebrow raised and ask you if you know how to make cough syrup because she has been having some chest congestion lately. That is when you can smile inside and have a quiet inner celebration.

how to treat the 12 common ailments

Here is a helpful guide on how to treat many of the common ailments that come up in most families. These remedies are gentle and safe, but be sure to test them out on yourself ahead of time to ensure you won't experience an adverse reaction.

Because many different plant medicines can be used in similar ways, it is useful to talk about general "actions" or properties. This way, you can find appropriate substitutes in case you don't have the specific ones I mention. For example, aloe vera and cactus are two entirely different species, yet they have very similar actions in the body. As you learn your local plants, start thinking in terms of "What action does this medicine have?" and you'll become wiser in how to use other plant medicines for similar conditions.

For all ailments, there are three very important universal aspects to healing: rest, hydration, and reflection.

The morning my leg was sliced open, I was dead tired from working too hard for the previous months. Exhaustion leads to accidents. When I've had chest infections, I see how I had been eating junk and rushing too much, which weakened my immune system and invited the trouble. Accidents and illnesses are nature's way to make you rest.

In addition, most people are severely dehydrated. Your body is 70 percent water and needs to move and flush things for healing processes.

And finally, there is always a greater lesson to be learned from ailments. They are gifts, in a strange sort of way. Honor them, and spend some time to find the meaning intended for you.

Bites, Stings, Rashes, and Burns

This first group of ailments is treated identically, so I'll discuss them together.

The actions you want for these ailments are cooling, soothing, drawing, and astringency. An astringent is an herb that has an action of tightening tissues and cells, and astringents help knit the body back together. Not surprisingly, it's a very common property in medicinal herbs, and about 60 percent of herbal medicines have some astringency.

Your initial focus when dealing with burns, bites, rashes, and stings is to cool them down. Ice is great for that, and if ice isn't available, cool water is another option. Flushing the area with cool water will help clean it, too.

When you've gotten the site cooled somewhat, apply a poultice made with one or a combination of the herbs that are cooling, soothing, drawing, and astringent. Here are some great materials to use that are widely available:

- **Aloe vera** (*Aloe barbadensis*) and prickly pear cactus (*Optunia* spp.). The inner meat of both plants has a nice, soothing, mucilaginous (also known as slimy), cooling, healing effect. Many people keep an aloe vera plant on their kitchen windowsill to have an immediate treatment for the occasional burn when cooking.

- **Clay.** Moisten dry clay with water, or mix it with aloe vera or cactus until you've got a nice, wet paste. Any clay you dig out of the ground will be fine. Black, red, orange—they are all good.

- **Plantain** (*Plantago major*). This is a common weed that grows everywhere. Use a bit of water and some fresh leaves, or a bit more water and dried leaves, and blend into a mush. Some people simply chew the leaves, mixing it with their saliva for the moisture. Apply as a poultice to the afflicted area.

- **Urine.** Back when I had allergies, I would have poison ivy outbreaks that were so severe my entire body was covered with weeping sores, and I couldn't sleep from the pain. The medicine I found to be most effective was my own urine. I drank lots of water, and when my bladder was full, I stood in the shower and slathered the urine all over my body, including areas that were not affected with sores. I let the urine soak on my skin for about 5 minutes and then I rinsed it off. I did this up to eight times a day. Urine is extraordinarily effective.

Cuts and Wounds

These remedies are for minor wounds and lacerations. If you have excessive bleeding and can't get it to stop, or if you have a head injury and have passed out, you definitely need more experienced health-care providers. These remedies are helpful with wounds from bruises, cuts, abrasions, lacerations, and early-stage infected wounds.

The actions you want for healing wounds are astringency, drying, drawing, styptic, antimicrobial, and vulneraries. The astringency helps with the inflammation. A styptic is an herb that helps stop bleeding. Note that the word "antimicrobial" includes antifungal, antibacterial, and antiviral properties. And vulneraries are herbs specifically known to be wound healers.

- **Honey.** Honey is an amazing wound medicine. After cleaning a wound, slather it with honey. Honey has antimicrobial properties, is soothing, and cleans and calms wounds. Be absolutely sure you've got a local, raw, pure honey, though. Most honeys sold in grocery stores contain little actual honey. And most honeys have been heated because it makes pouring and filling jars easier. Heat destroys the medicinal properties of the honey. If you can't afford raw, high-quality honey for eating, keep it around for wound care.

- **Plantain** (*Plantago major*). Plantain is soothing, cooling, astringent, antimicrobial, drawing, and styptic. Plantain has many different uses and is an abundant weed. Make a poultice of it like you do for bites and stings.

- **Yarrow** (*Achillea millifoleum*). Yarrow is the great styptic herb and is also antimicrobial and anti-inflammatory. Throughout history, even up until WWI, yarrow was the number-one remedy used on the battlefield to keep soldiers from bleeding to death. (The name "Achillea" is in honor of Achilles the great warrior.) On the battlefield, it was chewed and put directly on the wound.

- **Echinacea** (*Echinacea purpurea*). Effective in very serious situations such as a brown recluse bite or necrotic flesh, echinacea is well known for drawing poison out of the body. You'll need to have a tincture of it on hand for bites, and time is of the essence. Often with wounds from spider- or snakebites, the holes close up quickly due to swelling, and you'll want to get the tincture into the wound before it closes. If the flesh is becoming necrotic, apply a spray made from echinacea tincture, diluted with water by about half, to the affected area. Echinacea tincture should also be taken internally at the same time to fight internal infection.

- **Calendula** (*Calendula officinalis*). Calendula is a cousin of echinacea, but gentler. It fights the infection, soothes the wound, and helps the skin heal better. You'll see calendula is in almost every body-care salve or oil. It's just famous for helping the skin.

First, flush the wound with saline solution to remove any debris. Also remove any thorns, splinters, or stingers. Then, poultice the wound. Typically, you'll need to change the poultice every 4 hours.

Don't put oils or salves on these wounds in the early stages of healing. When they start to close later in the process, salves are fine.

With some deep puncture wounds, the wound near the surface heals more quickly and closes, trapping debris and potential infection deep in the punctured flesh. It isn't fun, but you may need to keep that puncture wound open until it heals from the inside out. Definitely have someone with more experience help you in this situation.

If you start to get fevers or spikes in fevers, get help from a trusted health-care provider. You should be seeing improvement within 2 days, but if not, seek help.

Coughs

You cough because something in your respiratory tract is irritated and it's not able to heal. Your lungs are unique to other organs in that they interface with the open environment through your breath (compared to your heart, liver, or other organs, which are all sequestered inside your body). Therefore, your lungs have greater exposure to outside irritants like pollen, air pollutants, or smoke. (Note that these remedies are not for chronic conditions such as asthma.)

One important question to ask is if the cough is dry or wet. A dry cough is raspy, and no phlegm comes out. Dry coughs are often much more spasmodic, sometimes uncontrollably so. For these, you need herbs with an antispasmodic action.

There is a bit of a double-edged sword with antispasmodics because you don't want to completely suppress a cough. You are coughing because your body wants to get something out, and if you try to completely suppress the cough, you are only going to drive it deeper into your lungs. The objective is to reduce some of the spasms and make the coughs more productive in getting more phlegm out.

For dry coughs, you want medicines that soothe, moisten, and loosen materials stuck in the lungs. And if the coughing could be helped by calming some of the spasms, adding some antispasmodics will help. Repeated dry coughing is also often very harsh on the throat, so you want a soothing action for the throat as well.

Wet coughs have mucus and phlegm, which may or may not be coming up, but you can hear it, that gurgling sound in the lungs and chest. Wet coughs are more prone to infection and could lead to walking pneumonia, so in addition to soothing, loosening, and an expectorant, you need a strong focus on antimicrobial action.

If the phlegm is yellow, green, or brown, an infection is present and you will definitely want antimicrobials. Probably several antimicrobials.

You can't do much about coughs without honey. Again, you are looking for a high-quality, local, raw honey. Honey by itself has many of the actions you want, including antimicrobial, antispasmodic, expectorant, and soothing. Honey is used as a base in all the cough medicines I've ever seen because it has so many of the actions necessary for helping coughs.

The honey in a cough syrup is immediately soothing to the throat, along with all its other properties, and the syrup's herbs are absorbed by the body and then excreted through the lungs. The lungs are intimately connected to the blood supply because that is how you take in oxygen and expel carbon dioxide. If you've ever had "garlic breath," you have firsthand experience of how herbs can be excreted through the lungs. That excretion through the lungs pushes out the irritants and helps the body fight infection.

As a worst-case scenario if honey just isn't possible to obtain, you can use sugar. Use one part sugar to one part medicinal tea. Make the tea out of herbs that contain the actions you are trying to achieve.

Here is a list of different herbs and some of their primary actions. Feel free to mix and match.

- **Elderberries** (*Sambucus nigra, Sambucus ebulus*). Elderberries are the foundational ingredient in classic cough syrup. They boost your immune system and reduce inflammation.

- **Mullein** (*Verbascum thapsus*). Mullein is a weed that grows all over the place, and the soft, big leaves and flowers are the medicine. It is highly regarded for helping the lungs and is good for dry, hacking coughs.

- **Ginger root** (*Zingiber officinale*). Ginger root is a really strong antispasmodic and antimicrobial. It's also anti-inflammatory, which helps with relieving pain.

- **Thyme** (*Thymus vulgaris*). Yes, this is the herb you probably have in your kitchen cabinet. It is antimicrobial and an expectorant and has a long history of being used to treat bronchitis and coughs.

If you are coughing really bad, take 1 teaspoon of homemade syrup every 30 minutes and then dial it down as you need.

If you have an infected wet cough with colored phlegm, you should be using antimicrobials internally, such as raw garlic, in addition to a cough syrup.

If the syrups, rest, hydration, and reflection aren't working, there is another option I've used: make a poultice of onions. It's very messy, but I've seen it prove effective for severe bronchitis. Chop at least two big onions into approximately ¼-inch pieces. Place them in a pot, just barely cover them with water, and simmer over medium heat until the onion is translucent. Add some cornmeal or other thickener to make a paste. With help, smear the paste on both the front and back of your chest and then wrap yourself in plastic wrap to hold it in place. Lie down, on a towel to limit the mess, for a half hour or so with a hot water bottle on your chest. Like I said, it's messy, but it's very effective. You may need to repeat the poultice, but you will definitely see some improvement with the first one.

Sore Throats

My favorite go-to remedy for a sore throat is numerous cups of warming, soothing, calming (uncaffeinated) herbal teas. The teas help keep you hydrated, moisten your throat, reduce spasms, and provide immune boosts with antimicrobial support.

My standard recipe uses licorice root (*Glycyrrhiza lepidota*) and slippery elm (*Ulmus* spp.) bark. Remember, the traditional slippery elm (*Ulmus rubra*) is in danger of overharvesting, so look for alternatives such as the elm tree in your backyard, or ask a local bioregional herbalist.

I just love this base recipe. Feel free to add other herbs you like, such as chamomile, lemon balm, peppermint, and honey.

The cough syrups mentioned earlier are also very helpful for sore throats.

Fevers

This might come as a surprise, but for the vast majority of fevers, the best thing to do is nothing. Well, keep yourself comfortable, warm, hydrated, and rested. But a fever is your body's natural system for healing and a response to some pathogens in your body. You are heating yourself to burn out the pathogen or inducing sweat to excrete the bad guys.

Many people immediately want to reduce a fever or make it go away, but this often interferes with the natural process your body wants to perform to take care of itself. You shouldn't interrupt it.

Let's set some parameters, though. If you (or a child over 8 years of age) have a fever over 102 degrees Fahrenheit for more than 2 days, or if you have an infant with a fever, definitely seek help from a trusted health-care provider. (Be sure you are accurately measuring with a thermometer you know works.) Also, if the fever comes with symptoms such as an unusual skin rash, persistent vomiting, or severe headache, you should seek outside help.

But for fevers lower than 102 degrees Fahrenheit, it's best to let them run their course. The body's best response to occasional pathogens is to burn them out with a fever.

It takes your body a lot of energy to heat up and maintain that high temperature. Many cultures use saunas or hot springs to proactively kill pathogens in the body. I often use a hot tub or sauna to raise or maintain a high core temperature, essentially using the external heat versus making my body produce all of it. This saves my body a lot of energy, so it can focus on excreting and healing. It also reduces the achiness that often accompanies a fever. If you don't have a hot tub or sauna, a pile of blankets works, too.

You also have to stay hydrated, so drink lots of broth and water. Part of the fever process is sweating out the pathogens, and you need to have lots of fluids to do this. Broths, and especially bone broths, are amazing medicines. Often you don't feel like eating, so broths keep hydration and nutrition coming in. You can also put some antimicrobial herbs into the broth. I find I often crave high-quality salts, too.

Don't forget the simple comforts of a cold cloth and the love of your family. I'll never forget one night when my daughter was very young. As she was sweating through a fever under a pile of blankets, I lay next to her with a cold cloth to wipe her forehead and cheeks. It was a tender time I know she appreciated and I now treasure.

Indigestion and Stomachaches

"Indigestion" is a vague term that encompasses nausea, acid reflux, flatulence, bloating, and swelling of the stomach or abdomen area. It's often caused by stress, improper eating habits (wolfing down food, eating while walking, not properly chewing, and so on), or eating food you are intolerant to. The vast majority of digestive problems come from eating too many refined carbohydrates, which cause inflammation of the gut.

This section is not meant to treat chronic or long-term problems. Also, if you have pain that radiates toward the lower-right quadrant of your abdomen, or if you have pains, swelling, or cramping near your liver (just under your right rib), go get help immediately.

These remedies are for those times when you ate too much Tex-Mex or if you want to improve your overall ability to digest food.

Bitter is both a flavor and an action in the body. It's also a taste lacking in the American diet. Bitters get your digestive juices flowing and are typically taken before or during a meal to prepare your system for the food coming in. Getting bitters can be as simple as eating some greens such as collards, arugula, or a fresh dandelion leaf or two. You don't need a lot. Those leaves, especially in the late summer, are nice bitters.

Carminatives are used to warm the digestive tract, get things moving, and dispel gas. Traditionally, many of the spices in ethnic foods weren't used necessarily for the taste, but because they help foods digest better. Carminatives are easy to add to your food, and you are probably already doing it. However, adding them with consciousness will improve their effectiveness. Some great carminatives to try are basil, anise, black pepper, caraway seeds, dill, cardamom, rosemary, cumin, and tarragon.

You know the little bowl of fennel seeds at Indian restaurants meant for you to grab and chew as you head home? Fennel is a great carminative, and this is why Indians have that tradition.

When you are really bloated and uncomfortable (for me, that's after eating too much wheat), ginger is an awesome warming, antispasmodic carminative.

Ginger is often used for nausea, too. Make a tea of it, or take some of the ginger syrup you hopefully prepared ahead of time. Note that fresh ginger is easier on the digestive tract.

You should not take bitters or ginger if you have some underlying hyper-secreting issue like ulcers. Also avoid these if you are pregnant or lactating. They definitely increase milk production (a secretion).

Ever wonder why after-dinner mints are so common? Mints (all of them in the *Mentha* spp.) are great digestion helpers.

If you have acid reflux or heartburn, a demulcent herb will be most beneficial. Demulcents are herbs that are soothing with an almost slimy quality. The most common demulcent is marshmallow, but hollyhocks, elm bark, and okra work, too. The leaves of the mallow plant also work, although the root is typically used. What you are looking for is a soothing, slimy tea that coats the internal mucosa of the intestines and calms everything. Unfortunately, the best demulcents are made in cold teas, which can take a few hours or even overnight. Some people who know they have digestive issues make a big batch ahead of time and leave it in the fridge.

Anxiety and Insomnia

Stress is characterized by an overactive nervous system. Herbal medicines can definitely help with stress, but some lifestyle changes are more beneficial.

Cut back on your consumption of negative media, including news, songs, websites, shows, and movies with violence, horror, and betrayal. Many years ago, I got into binge-listening to the folk trio Peter, Paul and Mary. After a while, I noticed I was getting depressed. One day I started really listening to the lyrics I was mindlessly repeating and realized that although the music was upbeat, the lyrics were depressing. When I changed the music, I felt a lot better.

I recently got an email that stated, "This information will both scare you and make you angry." I deleted the email immediately.

I'm not saying put your head in the sand and ignore what's going on, but focus on only letting in what's uplifting, inspiring, and happy, and your stress levels will go down.

Cut back on stimulants to your nervous system such as coffee and sugar.

In the hour before going to sleep, stay off your electronics. Read, stretch, make tea, brush your teeth, and calm yourself down instead. Be sure your bedroom is dark, with light-blocking curtains and any devices with LED lights unplugged or covered with black tape.

I absolutely depend on my meditation practices to help me stay in a good state of mind. There is a funny saying among meditators that you should meditate for an hour per day, except if you are really busy. In that case, you should meditate for 2 hours. It is true. You are much more efficient and productive with a peaceful mind.

Stress is often caused by mineral deficiencies, especially calcium, magnesium, and a group of other micronutrients. Because our food supply is so nutritionally impoverished, try some of the nourishing herbal infusions (page 229). The "big three" herbs with lots of calcium and magnesium are oats, nettles, and comfrey.

Milky oats (*Avena sativa*), which are the oat seeds harvested at the milky stage, are especially known for their calming effect on the nervous system. I recommend everybody try milky oats in teas, tinctures, syrups, or however you want to get them, on a daily basis.

Other plants with lots of micronutrients are common weeds. See Chapter 6 to learn which weedy species you can eat.

The act of making tea is a medicine in itself because it forces you to stop what you are doing, slow down, and drink a cup—hopefully with a friend. The leaves of the passionflower vine (*Passiflora incarnata*) make a wonderfully calming tea that is especially soothing to the nervous system.

Muscle Pain

You were out on the back 40 chopping firewood and now your muscles are really sore. Or maybe you strained something while lifting that heavy thing.

If the pain is sharp, acute, and strong, and you have an idea where it came from, it's likely muscle pain. That's the kind of pain I discuss in this section.

If the pain is dull, achy, and chronic, it's likely a joint-related issue. If the pain is a prickly hot feeling that is also almost numb, that is more likely a neural pain. The following remedies may help with these kinds of pains, but most likely you'll need some outside help from a chiropractor, sports medicine doctor, or other trusted health-care provider.

Like many conditions, it's best to approach muscle pain both internally and externally. The actions you want for both are warming, relaxing, pain-relieving, and antispasmodic. Some of the best herbs that fit this bill are black pepper, calendula, cayenne, chamomile, comfrey, echinacea, eucalyptus, ginger, lavender, myrrh, oregano, all the mints, and rosemary. For the internal support, you can simply make a wonderful spicy tea from a combination of some of these.

A great herb for the external application is a weedy species commonly called cedar trees or botanically anything in the *Juniperus* spp. These conifers grow almost everywhere, and you can use the needles to make a topically applied liniment, oil, or salve.

I know it's for horses, but I've often used Absorbine Veterinary Liniment for my own muscle pains. It's an herbal blend of calendula, echinacea, and wormwood.

All the liniments, oils, and salves are much better if they're applied and massaged in by a friend or family member.

A magnesium deficiency can cause achy muscles. Plants that contain lots of magnesium are chickweed, nettles, oat grass, and raspberry leaf. A magnesium supplement might also be helpful.

Soaking the affected parts in a warm bath of Epsom salt is a traditional way to soothe muscle pain. Epsom salt is high in magnesium, and your body will absorb some through your skin as you soak, which might be why this method has been successful for generations.

The bark of the willow family (*Salix* spp.), which includes cottonwoods, poplars, willows, and aspen, is calming, relaxing, pain-relieving, and antispasmodic. You make a tea from the bark, especially the bark of the younger twigs. Willow is called "nature's aspirin" and has been used as a pain-reliever for centuries.

Cannabidiol (CBD) oil is helpful for many. My friend Bonnie has enjoyed horses all her life. Now approaching her 70s, she has bruised, broken, and busted almost every part of her body numerous times. Bonnie swears by her homemade CBD salve. I'm not sure she could get out of bed without it.

Mucosal Injuries or Infections

The mucous membranes are the special sensitive inner linings of our skin: the nose, mouth, eyes, vagina, and rectum. They are all treated similarly, and because these areas are difficult to get to, you make an herbal wash to gently flush or saturate the area. It's a good idea to drink some of the wash to have the herbs working for you internally, too.

The mucous membranes are very sensitive areas, and many are right near the brain, so you need to be very careful about and proactive in getting outside help if the ailment isn't responding well to your home treatments.

The actions you are looking for are antimicrobial, soothing, cooling, anti-inflammatory, and mild astringency. Here are some herbs that help:

- **Calendula.** Calendula is very soothing, wound healing, and antimicrobial. It works especially well for hemorrhoids, yeast infections, and other vaginal infections. In Mexico, it is very common for dentists to send you home with a calendula mouthwash as part of your follow-up care after dental procedures.

- **Rose.** This beautiful flower is a very gentle astringent that helps bind proteins. It's very soothing for inflammation, only slightly antimicrobial, but very gentle, which is what you need for these delicate areas. In the commercial industry, roses are produced with a lot of pesticides, so do not use roses purchased from the grocery store unless they are grown organically. Fortunately, roses grow wild in many places.

- **Plantain.** Plaintain is an especially good antimicrobial and astringent, and it helps with inflammation. It also is a demulcent, which means it is soothing because of its kind of slimy property. It's especially good for nasal washes.

- **Lavender.** Lavender is a great herb and an especially strong antimicrobial.

The best way to use these plants is to make a wash out of one or a combination of a few.

When making the wash, use water that's as pure and clean as you have access to. The containers you use to mix and distribute the wash must also be as clean or sanitized as you can make them. Also, for every 1 cup of wash you make, add about ¼ teaspoon of salt so the mixture matches your body's natural salinity and is more easily accepted. Be sure to strain out the herbs before applying the wash.

You'll apply the wash three to five times daily. If possible, let the wash stay on for at least 5 minutes per session. For example, to treat an eye infection, tip your head back, fill your eye with the solution, and let the wash sit on your eye for a good 3 to 5 minutes for each of the three to five sessions per day.

Use an enema bag for the vaginal or rectal wash. A neti pot is helpful for nasal flushes.

chapter summary

- The plants make the medicine. We just arrange it into a convenient form.

- When using new medicines, always start with small doses and go slowly. Take the whole person into account, and adjust the dose and frequency if a person seems to need more or less.

- Experimentation, ritual, and intention are three secrets to unlocking the full power of herbs.

- Each herbal preparation has its own strengths and weaknesses.

additional resources

For more information on the eight preparations, check out these websites:

- https://Community.TheGrowNetwork.com. A very active forum where you can get any question answered about making and using herbal medicines from an experienced group of home medicine-makers.

- www.ElderberryCoughSyrup.com. An inexpensive kit to guide you in making your first syrup.

- www.HowToMakeATincture.com. Another inexpensive kit to guide you when making your first tincture. It includes the tincture bottle, the herbs, the recipe, and online support.

- www.MedicineMakingKit.com. Another inexpensive kit to guide you when making all eight preparations. It includes detailed video tutorials on how to make and use each medicine and a nice medical bag to store all your supplies in. I've had some difficulties sourcing the herbs, bottles, and pieces for this kit, so availability can be limited. All the kits are hand-assembled by my team of home herbalists.

chapter 9

herbal medicine in action:
my snakebite story

I was breaking the number-one rule in homesteading and in life: never put your hands or feet where you can't see them.

That's such a great rule, and it will keep you safe in so many situations.

I was barefoot and on my way to the tomato patch, which had grown into a huge jungle. I hadn't wanted that particular variety of tomato plants, but a freeze had wiped out my initial planting of the more orderly paste tomato bushes. Then my ducks had gotten into the next patch and sat on the second round of plantings. Every other gardener in the region had been hit by the freeze and was looking for replacement tomato plants, so the pickings were slim. Desperate, I bought the last ones the local garden center had.

I took extra-good care of those plants, feeding them well and encouraging what was turning out to be their megalomaniacal tendencies. They created a forest that sprawled and climbed all over everything. They were producing far more foliage than tomatoes.

But wow, did I start grinning when my explorations revealed a fat, 6-inch-diameter beefsteak tomato hanging in the shade. My mouth started to water as I cradled the heavy beauty. This tomato took two hands to hold and was perfect in symmetry, shape, and color.

I had no idea this thing had been growing in there. Oh, the bragging rights! It is almost impossible to grow a tomato this big in our climate, and nobody in their right mind tries growing beefsteaks. Growing a showcase specimen like this was a miracle.

Were there any more?

Recklessly I pushed into the nightshade jungle. That was my mistake. As I was almost to the middle, I felt the sharp sting from a cat's claw vine hook into the top of my foot. Reactively jerking my foot back, I felt the barb work its way in deeper.

On second thought, I realized there was a bigger problem. Cat's claw vines are common on my homestead, but there are no cat's claw vines, or any other plants with thorns, in my garden.

Hmm, was the sting from a really big scorpion?

Actually, it felt sort of like an ice pick in the top of my foot. It was stronger than a spider bite for sure. And it definitely hurt more than a fire ant bite.

Brushing aside the tangle of tomato plant branches, I knelt down and saw two neat puncture wounds in the top of my left foot and one big drop of blood. The three of them made a perfect equilateral triangle with about ⅜-inch sides.

The only thing that makes two punctures like that is a snakebite.

Rule One

The first rule of snakebite encounters is to stay calm.

Okay, I told myself, *I need to stay calm.*

I took a deep breath and went through the snakebite facts I knew.

The Centers for Disease Control and Prevention (CDC) states that venomous snakes bite only 7,000 to 8,000 people in the United States each year, and only about 5 of those people die.

I didn't really know those exact specifics at the moment, but I did know it was something like that. Anyway, I figured the odds were in my favor, and it helped keep me calm.

Rule Two

The second rule of snakebite encounters is to try to identify the snake.

You don't want to spend a ton of time doing this. Ideally, you should already know what snakes live in your area. Be familiar with what they look like so you can identify them quickly.

Hopefully, it was just a rat snake or a king snake, I thought. We have a lot of those guys because they like to eat my chickens' eggs. They also do valuable work eating mice and rodents in the barn, so I don't get too upset about them being around.

Plus, rat and king snakes aren't venomous. If one of them bites you, the worst thing that can happen is the wound gets infected. And preventing or treating infection is easy with good wound care.

So I would be happy if it were a rat or king bite.

Delighted, really, when you consider the other options.

In my area, the snake with the deadliest venom is the coral snake, with its bright red, yellow, and black bands. They look sort of like a corn snake, which is also occasionally seen in the area. To tell the difference between the two, remember that famous poem:

> **Red next to yellow, kill a fellow.**
> **Red next to black, okay for Jack.**

I do see the deadly coral snakes from time to time, but they are always very small. In fact, their mouths are generally too small to do much of anything to humans— except if they get a small toe or finger. But it is extremely rare in my area to get bitten—or die—from a coral snake.

Plus, the way this bite was on top of my foot, I knew it couldn't be a coral snake.

But I looked around under the tomato plants for the bright colors anyway, just in case. Even though I knew the likelihood of a coral snake biting me was low, a sigh of relief slipped out when I didn't see a coral snake anywhere.

I continued looking for any kind of snake.

The rattlesnake, for which the Southwest is famous, can certainly kill you, or at least make your life miserable for many weeks. According to Wikipedia, of the 20 venomous snakes in the United States, 16 are some form of rattlesnake.

But rattlers prefer rocky outcroppings, and I have never seen a rattlesnake on our sandy, post oak savannah land. None of my closest neighbors had ever mentioned seeing a rattler on their property either.

How do you know what kinds of snakes live in your area, especially if you have just moved in? Here are some suggestions:

- Start asking the neighbors. Everyone has snake stories. (You may hear more than you want to know, but at least you'll know what can be around.)

- Your local extension office, which probably has a wildlife biologist on staff, will also know.

- One of my favorite go-to wildlife books is the *Reader's Digest North American Wildlife*. This book is for all of North America, and there are lots of great books out there for your specific region. Look around, and I am sure you'll find one.

- And, of course, there is the internet.

The main takeaway is that it really is important to be familiar with the snakes, spiders, and other hazards that share your neighborhood.

I was pretty sure it wasn't a coral snake or a rattler. The other options were some of our more harmless snakes, like hognose or garter . . . or the final concern, a copperhead.

I knew that although a copperhead bite could also be a very painful experience—sometimes dragging on for weeks—it is rarely fatal. That's because people go get treatment right away.

Because I didn't see any snakes around, and I didn't want to spend a ton of time looking for the snake (and you shouldn't either), I walked back to the house.

My husband, Dave, was in the kitchen.

"I've been snakebit," I announced as I walked through the door.

"Do you know what kind?" he asked.

"No," I said.

He came over and looked at my foot. The drop of blood had smeared into a big Nike swoosh. He glanced up at the clock. "It's about seven forty-five—did it just happen?"

"Yes."

We both know it is good to keep track of the time and major events in any medical emergency. I knew Dave would start a record and be jotting things down.

"Does it hurt?" he asked.

"It is starting to," I said.

We both also knew what that meant. The only snakebite that would cause pain quickly was a copperhead.

He looked again. "Hmm, punctures about a quarter to three-eighths inch apart. . . . It was a young'un."

We both had heard the stories that baby copperheads are more dangerous because they can't control their venom and inject all they have when they bite. I don't know if that theory is true or not. And I guessed that although young, this one wasn't a baby.

But the venom in a young snake is just as dangerous as in a fully grown adult. The feeling of the fangs digging in when I jerked my foot back haunted me. I had probably gotten a good-sized dose.

"What should we poultice it with?" Dave asked. At this point, we had been married almost 20 years, and you don't need nearly as many words to communicate. He knew I would not go to the hospital.

He also knew the treatment would be to poultice my foot. Even though I thought I was still pretty clear-headed at that point, it is astonishing how reduced your mental capacity is in an emergency. That is such a good reason to have some plans in place ahead of time.

What should we poultice this with? I forced myself to focus on what would normally be a quick decision. I racked my brain to think of a good material. Being late June, the cabbages from the garden were long eaten and gone. We were way too far away from a store to get something quickly enough. Plantain is a good option at that time of year, but the plantain plants that grow on our land are very narrow-leafed and tiny. It would take forever to gather enough. Plus I didn't know if Dave could identify them.

I thought of the half-gallon jar of dried nettle leaf on the shelf in the pantry. But it wouldn't be enough, and I, in my getting-fuzzier state, wasn't totally sure that was a good poultice material anyway.

"Prickly pear pads," I said. "The ones behind the cowshed are a thornless variety and good sized." Why had it taken me so long to remember the prickly pear?

There really is no such thing as a thornless prickly pear, but some are less thorny than others.

Years ago, I saw a craigslist ad for free thornless cactus plants that needed to be rescued or they would be destroyed. A girlfriend and I made the expedition into Austin and filled two big sacks full of the pads. I planted them behind the cowshed, where it tends to be very hot and dry, which is what they like. I occasionally cut back the grass from around them, but they mostly thrived in their new home with little help from me. Over the years, they have given me much medicine and food.

I told Dave, "I am going to take a cold shower, and I'll be lying down here when you get back."

I pointed to the big rug. Everything of importance in our family happens either around the dining table or on the living room rug.

Every evening my family gathers around the rug to hang out together. Through the years, most of my kids' school projects were completed on the living room rug. Vast amounts of artwork have been created on the rug. Countless wrestling matches, yoga sessions, limbo contests, and gymnastics events have occurred on the rug. At Christmas, the wrappings covering piles of presents are ripped open on the rug. I birthed my daughter on the rug. (No, it has not been the same rug through the decades. With all that activity, we change it out every few years.)

Technically, I should have lain down immediately and skipped the cold shower. But I was hot and dirty from outdoor work, and I correctly guessed that things were going to get much worse. I didn't want to go into this experience sticky and smelly.

"Plus," I rationalized, "maybe the cold water will help slow my circulation."

Rule Three

The third rule of snakebite encounters is to lie down as soon as possible.

Dave took a long time to get the prickly pear pads. By the time he got back, my foot had swollen to my ankle, you could no longer see the puncture marks, and the pain was increasing.

It was definitely a copperhead bite.

Poulticing the Wound

If you recall, in Chapter 7, I wrote about having mastitis, a breast infection, when Ryan was a baby and how Dave and the midwife treated it with a poultice made of cabbage. Dave had never made a poultice out of prickly pear pads before, and he hadn't made another poultice since that breast infection. He knew the general principles, though, because he had seen me treat myself for other injuries. He is not the kind of guy to ask for or read directions, so he went at it boldly on his own.

He decided to skin the outside of a big pad and scar it "crisscross" with a knife to give it some flexibility. He attempted to apply this to my foot by tying it together with some cloth strips I keep in the medical bag.

I wondered if this technique might actually work.

It didn't.

Dave sort of understood it wasn't right and asked, "Is this okay?"

You certainly don't want to upset the people who are helping you in an emergency. I said, "Hon, I realize now why Doug always takes apart the pad to make a slimy mush for the poultice. That way the material can fit the contour of the body. The one you made doesn't get that much good contact." (Doug Simons is one of the many healers from whom I have learned about herbal medicines.)

Dave nodded with understanding while trying to work a small thorn out of his finger.

I casually mentioned that if you take two big rocks, you can use them to scrape all the thorns off the pad before removing the pad from the plant. It makes it super easy to harvest. And I have two rocks just for that purpose stashed by the back corner of the cowshed.

As he headed back out to the prickly pear patch, I asked Kimber to prepare some garlic for me. She nodded and understood that the garlic would help fight any internal infections. She peeled a fresh clove, crushed it with the side of a knife, and minced it. She brought me a tablespoon of the garlic mash medicine and a small glass of water as a chaser.

I wanted the garlic for insurance. I was about to ask her for some of the echinacea tincture when a wave of pain came. The echinacea would have been good to help my immune system, too. If the snakebite holes were still open, some people would put echinacea tincture right on the wounds, but with all the swelling, the holes were closed, and we were way past that.

And as events unfolded, I never got around to asking for the echinacea, and it was forgotten.

Poultice Attempt Two

Pain tends to come in waves, and it was rising quickly, coming in strongly, backing off a bit, and then surging to a new level of intensity.

With the next low in pain, I started giving Kimber directions on where to find the video on treating snakebites. Actually, the video is on how to treat all kinds of infections, broken bones, sprains, spider bites, and snakebites. The same treatment is used for all of them. When I created the video, I never dreamed it would be used in this way.

Dave came back from the prickly pear patch more quickly this time.

"How's the pain?" he asked.

We all laughed for a moment at the absurdity of that question.

Dave remembered the thing paramedics and doctors always ask: "On a scale of one to ten, how much pain are you feeling right now?"

That seemed funny, too. But we decided that a 1 or 2 was your typical fire ant bite or small scratch that drew some blood. Level 10 was so bad you were on the precipice of passing out. At about 5 or 6, the pain demanded most of your attention but was manageable.

I decided it was going in waves between a 3 and a 7. At its peaks, the pain absolutely demanded my full attention, but I had certainly endured worse.

Dave nodded agreement with my assessment. A copperhead had bitten him 3 years earlier, so he knew what I was going through.

Things started getting a little hazy for me as the waves came with more intense pain and less relief. When I came back from wherever I was going, I heard the sounds of chopping in the kitchen and the video going in the office.

Dave got a new, slushier version of the poultice on my foot. It felt so good. . . . The cool, slimy, green, soothing cactus was a good, good thing.

But there are two things about a poultice most people get wrong. The first mistake is that they make poultices too small. You really need to cover a large area.

When I surfaced from the next round of pain, I told Dave, "You know what, hon? We are going to need about four to five times more material. My whole foot needs to be encased in a poultice."

Dave went back to the patch again and got more pads. He came back much faster this time and made a bigger poultice.

At some point, I was vaguely surprised to become aware that both he and Kimber were in the office intently watching the video and figuring out what to do.

Dave discovered that he could use the blender to speed up the process of making the prickly pear slurry.

He also devised the following technique for applying the poultice to the unusually shaped area of my foot:

1. He put my foot into an old pillowcase.

2. He poured the prickly pear slurry in so it was covering and surrounding my entire foot, up past my ankle, and to my lower calf. (It takes a lot of plant material to do this.)

3. He used a plastic bag to contain the oozing coming out of the pillowcase.

4. He wrapped the whole thing with a towel and tied it in place with cloth strips.

The second mistake people make with poultices is that they don't keep them on long enough. You need to keep it on for hours, even overnight.

My Secret Painkiller

The pain was increasing. "Kimber," I called, "please get me that homemade pain medicine. It's in the far back of the pantry. The dark stuff in the pint jar with the white lid."

Normally, all my home medicine is labeled and dated. But this stuff is special, and only Kimber and I knew about it.

Dave furrowed his brow, "What is that stuff, hon?" he asked. "If I end up taking you to the hospital, I need to tell them. . . ." His words drifted off, but I knew what he meant. Our plan B would be to go to the hospital. You always need to have a plan B. Plans C and D are good, too. He would be watching me, and he knew I would give him a signal if I felt I was overwhelmed and could not handle the situation.

"It's a homemade painkiller made from prickly lettuce," I said. "It's nothing like the morphine they shot you up with. Don't worry, hon, it's legal; it's made from varieties of plants that are allowed."

Dave had been in such pain in the hospital when he was bitten. I had begged them to give him the morphine, even though it can cause a dangerous lowering of his blood pressure.

The homemade stuff I make wasn't strong enough to take away all the pain, and it doesn't affect blood pressure, but even just taking the edge off the pain is a really good thing sometimes.

I rarely used it, and when I did, it was because I really needed it. The prickly lettuce grows as a wild weed almost everywhere. It is pretty easy to grow it in your garden and process the medicine at home. I make a batch every few years so I always have a small supply on hand.

Kimber got me an ounce or so of the medicine.

I now was mostly focused on dealing with pain that was swinging more from five to eight on "the scale."

It was going to get much worse before the night was through. But every cloud has a silver lining, and in the coming agony, I would have a deeply life-changing mystical experience.

A Calm Voice in the Chaos

The pain was becoming loud. It was filling the room and bouncing off the walls. I began writhing on the rug. I sprawled this way and that, invisibly pinned down by my snake-bitten left foot.

I was groaning.

For a moment, Dave's blurry face loomed over me. His mouth was set in a line, and his eyes were studying me, searching for something. I tried hard to connect with his eyes, and I think I did briefly, to let him know I was all right.

I heard him rush back to the office where he and Kimber were still watching the video. I could hear their voices—Kimber, occasionally Dave, and mostly Doug Simons—as he explained in the video how traditional medicine worked. Their mottled sounds came to me, mixed in with the loudness of the pain.

I couldn't understand what they were saying.

I didn't care.

Suddenly, in the middle of the pain and the roaring in my ears, I felt a quiet, calm presence join me.

This presence was I, but not I. She was someone very familiar, very wise.

She pointed out that since I was writhing on the floor, why didn't I just go with it and proactively stretch my body?

I hadn't been to yoga in a few weeks, and I was pretty stiff.

It seemed like a good idea.

So I started to stretch and move my body ahead of the pain.

I stretched like I do on glorious, lazy Sunday mornings when I just take up the whole bed and twist and reach and move everything.

It felt good.

Really good.

As long as I kept it up, there was only the familiar release of muscles stretching. Pain yes, but a familiar pain, an easier pain.

A good pain.

She calmly explained that new elements of reality would come with this venom, and I needed to be flexible.

When I say she "explained"—it wasn't like I was hearing any words or seeing visions of anyone. I just had a strong sense that this was true. And the words I am writing here are my best attempt to explain what I understood at the time.

Many spiritual traditions and mystery schools have a name for this kind of encounter, including "your higher self," "guardian angel," or "spirit guide," to name a few.

I didn't see anyone or hear any words. I just "knew" things that are not a normal part of what I know.

I suppose you should always have some caution when dealing with this other layer of reality because other beings may not necessarily have your best interests in mind. But the suggestion to stretch had been a good one.

To an external observer, it may have appeared that I was flailing about on the floor. And seeing me so apparently out of control, I'm sure Dave and Kimber must have been anxious as heck. But internally, I was doing some really aggressive stretching.

Whatever. It was a good thing.

Shifting Resources

I don't know how long the intense stretching/flailing went on, but after a while, I felt my guts start to tremble.

The calm presence let me know my body could not afford to waste any resources on digesting the food I had eaten earlier, and it would have to go.

I called out, "Kimber, will you get me a big bowl, please?"

She brought the big stainless-steel bowl from the kitchen that we normally use for compost. I got up on my left elbow, leaned over the bowl, and retched.

The calm presence told me to breathe deeply.

I hadn't realized that, while I was vomiting, I was holding my breath.

I breathed deeply through my nose down to my root and was surprised to find how much more easily the remaining contents of my stomach came up.

For a moment, I again forgot to breathe, tightening involuntarily, and the retching was a painful struggle once more.

"Breathe," the calm presence reminded me.

I did, and again it felt miraculously easier.

In my life, I've had a few episodes of vomiting for one reason or another. And although this time wasn't exactly pleasant, it was the easiest I've ever had of it.

I rested for a while, surprised at this new insight.

Kimber took the bowl away, emptied it somewhere, and brought it back rinsed clean.

I went through two more long rounds of vomiting.

I was still in intense pain, and that and the loudness in my ears blocked most of normal reality. There was a pause here where I connected with the calm presence. I'm not sure how much time passed. I'll write it as best as I understand it, but again, it was not communicated in words or images, just through direct understanding.

She told me that the venom of a snake is an important gift.

If honored properly, it would mean big changes in my life. Most people are afraid of major changes, and that is the underlying cause of the deep fear many people have around snakes.

Unfortunately, she didn't have any specifics on just what changes would occur or exactly how I should honor the venom (although that would come later). I suppose the vagueness of the message is the problem with these kinds of encounters. But it was very reassuring, and it helped me relax into this whole process.

I had to agree with her that snakes have a really bad reputation that is largely undeserved. Adam and Eve immediately spring to mind whenever anyone says "snake." That story didn't exactly have a happy ending.

Physical reality came rushing back in with a new rudeness.

I discovered the contents of my colon had liquefied and needed to be released immediately.

It came out violently. Dave barely got me to the bathroom in time.

The convulsions for this release also came in waves over a period of time. The calm presence told me that this, too, was simply a part of the process. Like the contents of my stomach, what was in my bowels had to be gotten rid of. My body needed to focus its resources on healing and not on processing waste.

When this part was finished, it was well into the night. Dave helped me to bed. I lay down with the poultice sloshing around my foot and a pillow under my knee. The pain was just a throb down there—a very manageable 1 or 2 on the pain scale.

My body was empty, exhausted, and completely drained.

Before I drifted off to sleep, I felt the calm presence again.

Breathe

I understood that the way to honor the venom was to relearn to breathe deeply as an everyday, all-the-time thing.

Yes, yes, everyone takes a deep breath when they are stressed, and it is almost a joke to tell someone to take a deep breath when a situation starts to get out of hand. But seriously, if I would take on the challenge of actually breathing deeply as part of every moment of my life, many good changes would come.

She suggested I wear a bracelet. Every time I saw or touched the bracelet, I should remind myself to breathe deeply. The bracelet could be of any material, plain or colorful, simple or ornate, a gift or a purchase. It didn't really matter. The bracelet's primary function was to trigger a reminder to breathe deeply.

And in the mornings for a few minutes before I get out of bed, I should stretch like I had earlier that night. Maybe not quite as crazy. It could be done gently enough not to wake Dave if he were sleeping next to me. Just a few minutes' worth would be beneficial—like a cat waking from sleep.

Both of these suggestions made a lot of sense to me. Practical and simple, yet I could see that there would be profound benefits. I promised myself and "her"(?) that I would do these things and work to make them habitual.

Soon after that, I was fast asleep.

Recovery

I awoke late the next morning, my foot swollen and my mouth very dry.

Dave got me some water, and I gingerly began to drink. We opened the wrapping on my foot, wondering what my foot would look like. Dave joked that the prickly pear had slow-cooked through the night and smelled delicious.

It actually did smell good, and I am not sure he was completely joking. Overall, the swelling was slowly going down.

He applied a fresh poultice to my foot, with new wrappings.

To make one poultice, Dave told me he needed at least two big cactus pads. Each pad was about 10 or more inches in diameter and about ¾ inch thick. Prickly pear cactus grows almost everywhere on Earth, so you should be able to have a patch if you want to grow your own. It's definitely easier in hot, dry climates, but I've seen it growing in the tropics of Puerto Rico and the cold of Colorado.

And, as mentioned, many other plants work well, too.

I slept a lot that day. I wasn't that hungry, and I ate sparingly. To help rehydrate, I drank a lot of water, herbal teas, and some green juices.

The pair of crutches we keep by the medical kit came in very handy. I hobbled over to the office and did a bit of work on the computer, but mostly I stayed in bed, reading and sleeping.

I had no more vomiting, diarrhea, or even that much pain. My foot was swollen and tender, but there really wasn't much to say about it.

We kept my foot poulticed the entire day, changing it twice during the day and once more before I went to bed that night.

The following morning I felt much better. We took the poultice off for a few hours, and I could walk with only a bit of stiffness. I had Kimber drive the riding lawnmower over to the house, and I used that to get around and do my chores. This turned out to be really fun because I love any excuse to drive my zero-turn mower.

We had our annual project where we were growing out a big flock of chickens for meat. These chickens were not the usual heritage breeds I normally work with but rather Cornish rock crosses—"Franken birds" friends of mine jokingly called them. This breed is commonly used in commercial production, and they are somewhat unnatural creatures, so I was having to really adjust my systems to accommodate them. We had been having some unusual die-offs, which I think were due to the heat. But I was worried about them, and I was glad to be getting back to work.

When I came back to the house, we poulticed my foot for the day. But other than a few extra naps, I was mostly back to normal.

We had intended to poultice the foot that night, but I never got around to it. By the following morning, other than a bit of slight residual swelling and some tenderness, I was essentially as good as usual.

I had a meeting in Austin, and because the swelling was down, I comfortably wore a pair of shoes that were normally a bit big for me.

I am still amazed at the courage of both Dave and Kimber in handling this situation. Kimber was very knowledgeable in wild plants and plant medicines, but she was still very young. Dave had some experience, but he had never taken on a challenge that big alone. When Dave was bit by a copperhead, he wanted to go to the hospital for care, and I respected his choice.

But he knew that I had handled many other medical situations with natural medicines, and while I appreciate the existence of the medical system, it usually isn't my first choice.

No need to stir up trouble . . . unnecessarily.

In my mind, Dave is the real hero of this story for having the courage to take on a potentially life-threatening situation and trust his sometimes-difficult, definitely hard-headed wife.

Factors for Success

What factors enabled this story to have a happy ending? I count six key things:

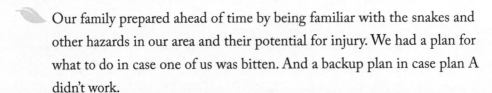 Our family prepared ahead of time by being familiar with the snakes and other hazards in our area and their potential for injury. We had a plan for what to do in case one of us was bitten. And a backup plan in case plan A didn't work.

I have used traditional medicine for many years. I know the process for making and using these treatments. I have experienced amazing healing on many other injuries, both big and small, and I trust myself to use them well.

I have a good sense of knowing what I can handle and when I should call for outside help (as in going to the hospital). And yes, knowing that the medical system is there as a backup is reassuring.

I have a strong immune system from years of eating good food, exercising, and taking care of myself. My body is strong and flexible and has excellent reserves. I trust my body to heal.

We had a good supply of medicines on hand.

Most importantly, my family is very supportive, knowledgeable, and willing to care for me.

As in many families, I am the one with most of the medical skills, so having the resources for them to watch and refer to was very useful. Historically, families kept a big book with details of medical events and how they treated them—both successfully and unsuccessfully. What a treasure that would be to pass down through the generations! Wouldn't you like to know what ailments your ancestors had and how they dealt with them? It could be so useful and revealing about issues you are challenged with today.

But let's be clear: if you get bitten by a snake and you want to try and handle it yourself, you need to have all these important pieces in place ahead of time.

Please don't think you can just wing it. The low number of deaths from venomous snakebites is because people seek treatment right away.

I hope this story empowers you to start taking some of those steps. You can grow this.

I am writing my story as an example of the surprising benefits of true wealth. I could not have done this without my great health, my family, and the community of healers I've known over the years. Amazing things are possible as you grow.

chapter summary

- Get to know the hazards in your area—what snakes, spiders, animals, or venomous insects share the earth with you? What do they look like? Where do they commonly live?

- Have a plan and a backup plan. Know when you need to call in help.

- Start making and using traditional medicine on small ailments or injuries.

- Work on improving your general health, especially your immune system, by eating deeply nutritious foods and staying active.

- Involve your family, friends, and community because we all need each other at some time in our lives.

additional resources

For more information on treating infections and boosting your immune system, check out these websites:

- www.TreatingInfections.com. The video I created with Doug Simons with step-by-step directions for treating infections without antibiotics. It covers snakebites, stings, lacerations, sprained and broken bones, and more. It also includes lots of information on poulticing, materials, and supporting herbs to take internally.

- www.HomemadePainkiller.com. A free ebook on how to make an effective homemade painkiller from wild lettuce.

- www.ImmuneBoostingHerbs.com. A free series of reports on deeply nutritive herbs you can take regularly to boost your immune system. The reports include the history, dosages, uses, parts of the herb, best preparations, identification tips, growing advice, and lore.

- www.7DaySugarChallenge.com. The biggest thing you can do to strengthen your immune system is to cut back the amount of sugar you eat. This free series of emails gives you my best tips, tricks, and techniques to quit sugar.

safeguard your family, now and **for the future**

real nutrition: why you need it and how to get it with **nutrient-packed infusions**

A mysterious epidemic raged in the American South during the first part of the early 1900s. The illness was characterized by a progressive series of symptoms, starting with skin rashes, lesions, a swollen tongue that turned black, diarrhea, mental problems, and then death. Because so many people were sick and dying, speculation about the cause of the disease was intense and rampant. Was it the black, disease-transmitting Simulium flies? Yellow fever and malaria had been traced back to insects, so it seemed plausible that this, too, was an infectious disease carried by flies. Or was it transferred by kissing or touching? Was it evil spirits?

Rural southerners tend to be prone to superstition more than those from other areas of our country. (I can attest to this, being a born-and-bred southerner.) You can only imagine the other possible explanations, and remedies, that were created to explain this horrible malady.

The biggest clue to the surprising conclusion of the epidemic was . . . corn.

The disease, later identified as pellagra, mostly affected people who were living on subsistence diets that relied heavily on corn for calories. The biggest outbreaks of the disease came in the summertime, when corn consumption was the highest. But corn was a staple crop cultivated and eaten for thousands of years by the indigenous people of what we now call Mexico and Central America. They didn't have any disease issues using corn as a staple in their diet. What was the difference?

The American southerners enthusiastically embraced crops of corn because it was so much more productive than rye or other grains. But they did not adopt the ancient techniques developed by indigenous peoples for processing the corn. How these ancient peoples knew to soak their corn in an alkali solution (made from lime) is an astonishing mystery. This process, known as nixtamalization, helps release more nutrients from the corn kernels, and especially the nutrient vitamin B_3, also known as niacin.

Dr. Joseph Goldberger was a physician who heroically proved that pellagra was caused by a nutritional deficiency of vitamin B_3. When processed correctly, corn releases vitamins, but it can cause a nutritional deficiency if it's central to a diet and has not been soaked. His struggle was against the prevailing medical belief system that insisted disease was primarily caused by germs. Dr. Goldberger had to repeatedly prove that a nutritional deficiency was the culprit. Interestingly, instead of adopting the traditional processing of the grain to release the vitamins in corn, they ended up adding brewer's yeast to people's diets because it is high in B vitamins, especially niacin.

Many Traditional Ways of Preparing Food Are Based on Maximizing Nutrition

Our elders have an astonishing amount of wisdom about how to prepare foods to maximize nutrition. One of my favorite cookbooks is *Nourishing Traditions: The Cookbook That Challenges Politically Correct Nutrition and the Diet Dictocrats* by Sally Fallon. Sally's book shows how modern people can bring back some of these traditional food preparation methods that maximize the food's nutritional value, and includes delicious recipes. Many people don't realize that we are wired to seek out more nutritious food because it often tastes better. This is yet another way that nature provides—flavor and nutrition go hand in hand.

One time, Sally and I were doing an interview and I went off-topic on a tirade about how overprotective today's moms are. I remember saying, "Sally, I never wore helmets and elbow pads just to ride a bike. I don't know why moms have to cover their kids with all this safety gear." Sally quickly interjected and told me that today's moms are absolutely right in insisting on extra safety gear. She explained that when I was growing up, there was more nutrition in the common food supply. But the nutrients have been steadily dropping over the decades, especially when it comes to the calcium needed for healthy bones. Studies show that the skulls of kids born today are thinner than in previous generations, and the rates of concussions, skull fractures, or breaks are much higher.

In addition, the CDC predicts that one out of every three children born in 2000 will become diabetic. Everyone points to this huge increase as a result of lifestyle choices. The focus is on movement and exercise, which are important, but malnutrition is a much larger factor in our declining health and the declining health of our children.

Where Did All the Nutrition Go?

Because our soils have become depleted, the food most of us eat isn't packed with nearly the amount of nutrients it could be. In basic terms, this means today's supermarket carrot just isn't as good for you as the carrots your grandparents ate. One of the largest and most compelling studies on this topic was published in 2004 in the *Journal of the American College of Nutrition*. Using data from the archives of the U.S. Department of Agriculture (USDA), a team of scientists looked at the nutrient content of 43 fruits and vegetables grown in 1950, everything from rutabaga to honeydew, and compared them to the identical fruits and veggies grown in 1999. Their findings were disturbing—all the nutrient levels went down. Not a single nutrient had increased in the past 50 years.

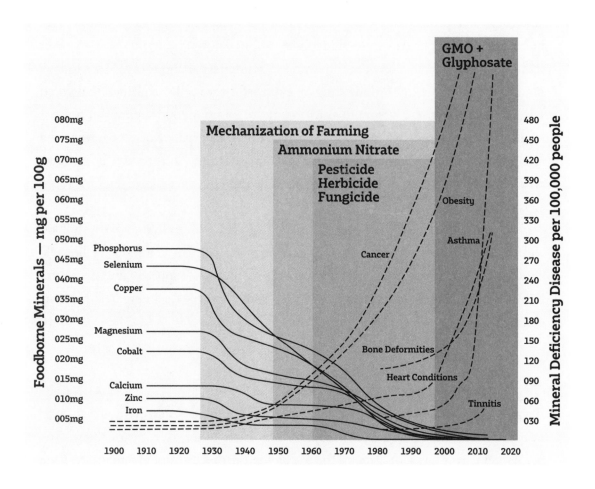

Our country cannot have a meaningful conversation about reforming the health-care system until the quality of our food supply is addressed.

If you feel sluggish, are often sick, have trouble sleeping, crave sugar, or have fuzzy thinking, you are likely undernourished. A lack of proper nutrients also puts you at a higher risk of cancer, diabetes, heart disease, and chronic obstructive pulmonary disease (COPD). I know that sounds scary, but frankly, you should be concerned. Nutrient deficiency is always associated with these diseases. Ironically, undernourishment is also one of the primary reasons for our nation's obesity epidemic. Our food has plenty of calories, but it's virtually devoid of nutrients. Our bodies crave those nutrients, but we give them empty calories. So the cravings continue. We eat and eat, growing fatter each year, but we never give our bodies what they really need and satisfy our true hunger. It's a self-reinforcing pattern—a trap.

By the way, the flipside of this is wonderful. If your body is stocked full of all the nutrients it needs, your food cravings will diminish. You can actually follow your appetite, instead of fighting it.

Can Dietary Supplements Fill the Nutritional Void?

Look through almost anyone's kitchen cabinets, and you'll likely see a collection of white plastic bottles with vitamin C tablets, vitamin D_3 gel caps, and an assortment of other supplements. At some level, I think we all understand that we aren't getting the nutrition we need from the commercial food supply. A friend of mine is a divorced dad who is deeply concerned about the food his ex is feeding the kids. He gives his children high-quality multivitamins when he has them and hopes for the best. He shrugged his shoulders and told me he is not sure if they do any good, but it's all he can do to try to help in a situation he can't control.

Dietary supplements composed an estimated $115 billion global industry in 2018. Practically everyone has used vitamin and/or mineral supplements at some point in their life, if not on a regular basis. And why not? After all, it's really easy to just pop by your local drugstore, pull one of the many offerings off the shelf, and feel like you're doing something good for your health. But are you?

From time to time, I totally get swept up in the supplements craze. I'll read a study about something that points to a deficiency in, say, selenium, and I'll worry if I have enough selenium in my body. I'll run out and buy the highest-quality selenium supplement I can find and hope I've got that nutritional base covered. But is it really a good idea to take pure selenium? There is nothing like that out in nature. . . .

There are definitely people who have been helped with nutritional supplementation, especially when they are working with a skilled health-care practitioner. But it is tricky. Here is just one example of how complex effective supplementation can be. For years, women over 50 were told to take calcium supplements. But did you know that you should not take calcium carbonate because it has a hard time being absorbed in older bodies? Instead of going into a person's bones, calcium carbonate may get absorbed in artery walls, leading to the hardening of the arteries, heart disease, and stroke. On the other hand, calcium citrate *can* be absorbed by the body, but only if you are taking it with the proper amount of magnesium to help with absorption. Oh, and you also need to take some vitamin D with it, too. *Whew!*

That's a lot of information to be aware of and balance if you want to safely take just one of these common supplements.

Where Do Supplements Come From?

Ninety percent of vitamins are synthetic, even the ones labeled as "natural" or "food-based." Yes, even the expensive ones at your local vitamin stores, membership clubs, or health-food stores are often synthetic. There are some great reputable supplement companies out there. But the truth is, many vitamin brands are manufactured by a handful of large pharmaceutical companies and just packaged in different containers for marketing purposes.

But does that really matter? Is a synthetic vitamin really any different from one you'd find in nature? Absolutely! There's not just one form of vitamin D or vitamin C. Vitamins come in many different forms. As I discussed in Chapter 8, a humble medium-sized apple has only 5 mg of vitamin C, but it has the antioxidant impact of a 1,500 mg tablet of ascorbic acid synthesized in a lab.

Regardless of how modern we are, our bodies are built with a template that expects our nourishment to come from foods grown in nature. We are designed to absorb and use nutrients that come in the complex packages of fruits, nuts, meats, and vegetables. Synthetic vitamins are in forms that are isolated and alien to our biology. Often, they're produced synthetically from petroleum-based chemicals in manufacturing plants.

Not only are synthetic vitamins less beneficial, they can be actively harmful. Your body often treats these synthetic vitamins as foreign substances (because they are) and launches an immune response against them. This can lead to cascading problems down the line.

Mineral supplements aren't much better. Most of these are obtained through mining, derived from rocks such as limestone, coral, sand, and chalk. Technically, they have the same mineral profiles as the minerals we need, but our bodies weren't designed to digest and absorb rocks and are very inefficient at doing so. These petroleum- and mining-based supplements do have one advantage over plant-based supplements, though. They're much cheaper to produce on a commercial scale. This means they can outcompete any company that really wants to make a quality supplement. The financial incentive is very much against good supplements.

Are You Overnourished?

Gaining nutrition through supplements, as opposed to through food, can pose other risks. When you eat food, your body's cravings can guide you to the nutrients you need and away from the ones you don't. But supplements don't allow that level of discrimination. Maybe you need more calcium. Maybe you don't. But if it's in the supplement, you'll be getting it either way.

Why does that matter? Because excesses of certain nutrients can cause just as many problems as deficiencies. For example, calcium supplementation has been shown to actually increase the risk of hip fracture. And people taking calcium supplements are at a higher risk of death from cardiovascular disease. Calcium supplements can also inhibit the uptake or iron, some studies showing by as much as 62 percent.

On the other hand, if you're eating calcium-rich foods, you are unlikely to build up unsafe levels of calcium in your body. Your cravings will change and steer you to different foods. Your body is amazing at keeping a balance of nutrients, if you listen to it. And, as in the earlier apple example, the calcium in whole foods comes packaged with other nutrients your body expects.

Pill-based supplements don't give you this option. Unless you're getting regular blood tests to monitor your nutrient levels, you're basically just guessing.

The Big, Dirty Secret of "Organics"

This may come as a surprise to you, but although eating organic may help you reduce your exposure to antinutrients such as pesticides, herbicides, hormones, and

GMOs, organic foods *do not* contain any more nutrition than conventional produce. Stanford University analyzed 237 studies of organic produce, meats, and dairy foods and concluded that organic foods are no more nutritious than their conventional counterparts. (Read the analysis for yourself here: https://med.stanford.edu/news/all-news/2012/09/little-evidence-of-health-benefits-from-organic-foods-study-finds.html.)

Also, as organic production has become industrialized, the quality has dropped significantly. Dr. Phillip Howard is a member of the International Panel of Experts on Sustainable Food Systems. Dr. Howard has been monitoring the organic industry for several decades and has noted that as large corporations have bought out smaller organic brands, the quality of the products has often been sacrificed. So even if you are buying all-organic ingredients, you are likely still not getting enough nutrition from your food.

How Do You Supplement Your Nutrition While You Create Your Grow System?

A deeply nourished body is your greatest form of wealth. The primary way you can achieve this is by growing and eating your own food. That really is the ultimate way to get your nutrition.

As discussed in Chapter 5, your soil is truly the best source of your nutrition. That is the primary reason I recommend raised beds—it's the best way to help you focus on what is really important, and that is the life and vibrancy of the bit of earth where you are growing your food supply. And as discussed in Chapter 6, foraging for wild edibles is another source of nutrition, but that also takes a bit of time to learn, and of course, we don't want to overharvest.

It does take time to get these systems up and running and develop the skills to really reach this level of self-sufficiency. The good news is that there is a simple and easy way to get the nutrition you need right now. And you can continue to use this method to boost your health when you have your grow system running, too. Throw out those multivitamins—herbal infusions are all you need!

Good Nutrition Fast: The Five Nutrient-Packed Infusions

"You can drink your way to health," says Susun Weed, founder of the Wise Woman School of Herbal Medicine. Susun is the undisputed expert on using nourishing herbal infusions to increase your nutritional levels and up your health quotient. Susun has been drinking nourishing herbal infusions for decades, and at 76 years old, she is still sharp, clear, and full of energy.

If you recall from Chapter 8, an infusion is similar to an herbal tea, except you use a lot more herb and let it brew for a lot longer. An herbal infusion uses approximately 1 ounce of herb by weight, or for most herbs, that translates to 1 heaping cupful by volume. That is a lot of herbal material. And that is part of why these nourishing infusions are so effective.

Almost all herbs have nutritional components, but there is a special category of herbs known as "nutritional herbs" that are perfect for making nourishing herbal infusions. To make it into this special category, an herb needs to be deeply nutritious, have insignificant undesirable components, and be safe to consume in large quantities on a regular basis. They are whole, complete foods that are loaded with nutrients easily absorbed by the body. But the most important characteristic is that they taste good. There are lots of super herbs loaded with nutrition that are safe in large quantities, but honestly, they taste awful and no one will drink an infusion made with them.

As I mentioned, you need to take a big quantity of these herbs, and they need to be prepared in a special way. The process is simple, though—as easy as making iced tea.

But first, let me introduce you to five supercharged nutritional herbs that work best for infusions. I was completely shocked when I first saw how much nutrition was packed into these special herbs. It made me rethink everything I knew about getting nutrition. It's incredible that it is really this easy to give your body a powerful, truly all-natural and effective supplement.

nutritional profile*

oat straw

	Trace	Very Low	Low	Avg.	High	Very High	Per 1 oz.	RDA% per 1 oz.
Aluminum	▨						trace mg	N/A
Ash (total)	▨▨▨▨▨▨						2.32 mg	N/A
Calcium	▨▨▨▨▨▨▨						405.40 mg	31%
Calories	▨▨▨▨▨						20 cal	1%
Chromium	▨▨▨▨▨▨▨						0.11 mg	N/A
Cobalt	▨▨▨						0.05 mg	N/A
Crude Fiber	▨▨▨▨▨						4.90 mg	N/A
Dietary Fiber	▨▨▨▨▨						17.58 mg	N/A
Fat	▨▨▨						19.84 mg	0%
Iron	▨▨▨▨▨						0.38 mg	2%
Magnesium	▨▨▨▨▨▨▨▨						340.19 mg	81%
Manganese	▨▨						0.01 mg	1%
Niacin	▨▨▨▨▨▨▨						2.13 mg	13%
Phosphorus	▨▨▨						79.66 mg	6%
Potassium	▨▨▨						77.11 mg	2%
Protein	▨▨▨						2.04 mg	N/A
Riboflavin	▨▨▨▨▨						0.06 mg	4%
Selenium	▨▨▨▨▨						0.04 mg	67%
Silicon	▨▨▨▨▨▨▨						0.52 mg	N/A
Sodium	▨▨▨▨▨▨▨						111.13 mg	5%
Thiamine	▨▨▨▨▨						0.06 mg	5%
Tin	▨▨▨						0.17 mg	N/A
Vitamin A	▨▨▨▨▨▨▨						3401.94 IU	68%
Vitamin C	▨▨▨▨						3.4 mg	4%
Zinc	▨						trace mg	0%

*Nutritional information sourced from Nutritional Herbology: A Reference Guide to Herbs (Pederson, Mark. Warsaw, IN: Whitman Publications, 2010).

Oat Straw (*Avena sativa*)

I remember the first time I learned that straw is packed with nutrients. I couldn't believe it. I mean it's just oat *straw* . . . what could possibly be in that? But the amount of magnesium alone tells the story. Oats, both the tops and the straw, historically have been known to be very soothing and calming. Both parts also are high in magnesium, which is an essential mineral for nerve function.

Oat straw has a mild, salty flavor and a cooling, moistening energy. It's a great restorative and strengthener for the whole body. But it has a special affinity for the nervous system. Oat straw will help clear your mind and soothe stressed, frazzled nerves. It has a mood-lifting effect and is reputed to support sexual health as well. As a side effect of its soothing nature, oat straw has pain-relieving qualities for the whole body.

Check out the nutrition in oat straw.

Nettles (*Urtica dioica*)

Nettles are the powerhouse of nutritional support. Nettles have a slightly salty taste and a drying, cooling energy. Nettles help your body respond better to stressors, assist with detoxification, support boundless energy, and generally move your entire body from a state of sickness toward a state of health. Nettles also have a strengthening effect on bones and connective tissues. It's one of those rare herbs that seems to help with just about everything.

Yes, these are stinging nettles, but don't worry. The sting disappears when they are dried. If you're growing or wildcrafting your own, wear gloves when you harvest them.

nutritional profile*

nettles

	Trace	Very Low	Low	Avg.	High	Very High	Per 1 oz.	RDA% per 1 oz.
Aluminum	/////						3.91 mg	N/A
Ash (total)	/////////						2.38 mg	N/A
Calcium	////////////////////////						822.14 mg	63%
Calories	/////////////						17.01 cal	1%
Chromium	///////////////////////						0.11 mg	N/A
Cobalt	///////////////////						0.37	N/A
Crude Fiber	////////////////						3.12 mg	N/A
Dietary Fiber	////////////////						12.19 mg	0%
Fat	////////////////						.65 mg	0%
Iron	////////////////						1.19 mg	7%
Magnesium	//////////////////////						243.81 mg	58%
Manganese	//////////////////						0.22 mg	10%
Niacin	////////////////						1.47 mg	9%
Phosphorus	//////////////////						126.72 mg	10%
Potassium	/////////////////						496.12 mg	11%
Protein	//////////////////						7.14 mg	N/A
Riboflavin	//////////////////						.12 mg	9%
Selenium	//////////////////						0.06 mg	113%
Silicon	//////////////////						0.29 mg	N/A
Sodium	//////						1.39 mg	0%
Thiamine	///////////////						0.15 mg	13%
Tin	////////////////						0.76 mg	N/A
Vitamin A	//////////////////						4450.87 IU	89%
Vitamin C	//////////////////						23.53 mg	26%
Zinc	///////////////////////						0.13 mg	1%

*Nutritional information sourced from Nutritional Herbology: A Reference Guide to Herbs (Pederson, Mark. Warsaw, IN: Whitman Publications, 2010).

nutritional profile*

red raspberry leaf

	Trace	Very Low	Low	Avg.	High	Very High	Per 1 oz.	RDA% per 1 oz.
Aluminum							11.1 mg	N/A
Ash (total)							2.27 mg	N/A
Calcium							343.03 mg	26%
Calories							16 cal	1%
Chromium							0.04 mg	N/A
Cobalt							0.1 mg	N/A
Crude Fiber							2.32 mg	N/A
Dietary Fiber							9.16 mg	0%
Fat							0.48 mg	0%
Iron							2.86 mg	16%
Magnesium							90.43 mg	22%
Manganese							4.14 mg	180%
Niacin							10.83 mg	68%
Phosphorus							66.34 mg	5%
Potassium							379.88 mg	8%
Protein							3.20 mg	N/A
Riboflavin							trace mg	0%
Selenium							0.07 mg	129%
Silicon							0.04 mg	N/A
Sodium							2.18 mg	0%
Thiamine							0.1 mg	8%
Tin							0.62 mg	N/A
Vitamin A							5375.92 IU	108%
Vitamin C							104.04 mg	116%
Zinc							trace mg	0%

*Nutritional information sourced from *Nutritional Herbology: A Reference Guide to Herbs* (Pederson, Mark. Warsaw, IN: Whitman Publications, 2010).

Red Raspberry Leaf (*Rubus idaeus, Rubus strigosus*)

Red raspberry leaf has a pleasantly fruity, sour taste. It's cooling and drying by nature and has an overall balancing effect on the body. It helps reduce inflammation throughout the body and can assist in blood sugar management. It is famous as a women's herb, because it helps to tonify the uterus. Pregnant women, or women with menstrual cramps, often find relief and support by drinking raspberry leaf tea.

Harvest raspberry leaves after you harvest your raspberries but before the leaves drop. They are a whole second crop from your bushes.

Comfrey Leaf (*Symphytum officinale*)

Comfrey leaf has a mildly sweet-and-salty flavor and imparts a moist, cool energy. Much like oat straw, comfrey has a soothing and lubricating effect across the body. It helps relieve sore, tight muscles and arthritis pain, but comfrey's main claim to fame is its ability to heal wounds. Comfrey stimulates the healing systems of the body in a big way—more than any other herb.

nutritional profile*

comfrey leaf

	Trace	Very Low	Low	Avg.	High	Very High	Per 1 oz.	RDA% per 1 oz.
Aluminum							6.72 mg	N/A
Ash (total)							1.02 mg	N/A
Calcium							510.29 mg	39%
Calories							17.01 cal	1%
Chromium							.05 mg	N/A
Cobalt							trace mg	N/A
Crude Fiber							2.55 mg	N/A
Dietary Fiber							13.61 mg	0%
Fat							0.34 mg	0%
Iron							0.34 mg	2%
Magnesium							19.84 mg	5%
Manganese							0.16 mg	7%
Niacin							2.52 mg	16%
Phosphorus							62.37 mg	5%
Potassium							481.94 mg	10%
Protein							3.97 mg	N/A
Riboflavin							0.20	16%
Selenium							0.03 mg	62%
Silicon							0.26 mg	N/A
Sodium							3.12 mg	0%
Thiamine							0.06 mg	5%
Tin							0.19 mg	N/A
Vitamin A							5102.91 IU	102%
Vitamin C							22.68 mg	25%
Zinc							trace mg	0%

*Nutritional information sourced from *Nutritional Herbology: A Reference Guide to Herbs* (Pederson, Mark. Warsaw, IN: Whitman Publications, 2010).

nutritional profile*

red clover blossoms

	Trace	Very Low	Low	Avg.	High	Very High	Per 1 oz.	RDA% per 1 oz.
Aluminum							3.88 mg	N/A
Ash (total)							1.28 mg	N/A
Calcium							371.38 mg	29%
Calories							19.84 cal	1%
Chromium							0.09 mg	N/A
Cobalt							0.05 mg	N/A
Crude Fiber							2.81 mg	N/A
Dietary Fiber							10.21 mg	0%
Fat							1.02 mg	0%
Iron							trace mg	0%
Magnesium							98.94 mg	24%
Manganese							0.17 mg	7%
Niacin							3.54 mg	22%
Phosphorus							91.29 mg	7%
Potassium							566.99 mg	12%
Protein							3.26 mg	N/A
Riboflavin							0.09	7%
Selenium							0.02 mg	41%
Silicon							0.03 mg	N/A
Sodium							4.54 mg	0%
Thiamine							0.12 mg	10%
Tin							0.71 mg	N/A
Vitamin A							569.26 IU	11%
Vitamin C							84.08 mg	93%
Zinc							trace mg	0%

*Nutritional information sourced from *Nutritional Herbology: A Reference Guide to Herbs* (Pederson, Mark. Warsaw, IN: Whitman Publications, 2010).

Red Clover Blossoms (*Trifolium pratense*)

Red clover blossoms have a sweet taste and pleasant aroma. Like red raspberry leaves, they have a special affinity for women's health issues, but they can also have beneficial effects on prostate health. Red clover likes to clear up skin issues and strengthen bones. It runs through the veins, keeping them clean and improving circulation. It's also fond of keeping the respiratory and digestive systems functioning correctly. Red clover is a real multitasker.

You can grow these nourishing herbs at home, wildcraft them, or buy them in bulk—whichever works best for you. Comfrey and nettles are considered invasive weeds and can be found in many places. Oats are super easy to grow and thrive just about everywhere. Raspberry leaf is the byproduct of growing raspberries. Red clover blossoms? Well, those are definitely harder to get in quantity. But as you can see, many of these herbs are easy to obtain or cultivate.

Here are some other great candidates Susun recommends for nourishing herbal infusions:

- Linden flowers (*Tillia americana*)
- Chickweed (*Stellaria media*)
- Mullein stalk and leaf (*Verbascum thapsus*)
- Hawthorn berries, leaves, and flowers (*Crataegus* spp.)
- Elderberries or flowers (*Sambucus canadensis*)
- Burdock root (*Arctium lappa*)
- Violet leaves (*Viola* spp.)
- Plantain leaves (*Plantago* spp.)
- Marshmallow root (*Althea off.*)
- Slippery elm bark (*Ulmus fulva*)

Making Infusions

Making an infusion is so easy, you will wonder why you've never heard of it before. It takes only a few minutes. Here is my routine for making sure this happens every day.

First, I put some water on the stovetop to boil. My favorite time to do this is in the evening, just before I brush my teeth. I am the kind of person who absolutely needs to have a teakettle that sings when it's boiling. I am so easily distracted by emails, the phone, the dogs barking at something, or the chickens disturbed. I've got to have a loud reminder, and a pot that sings is just the remedy.

After I've filled up the teakettle, I take a heaping cup or more of dried herbs (as much as a cup and a half—remember, nature is not nearly as fussy as computers) and put it in a quart-sized canning jar.

While the water is heating, I go brush my teeth. By the time my teeth are clean, the water will be ready. I pour the boiling water over the herbs, stir them for a moment, and loosely cover the jar.

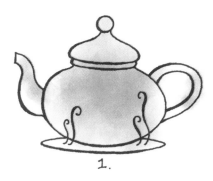

1.

PUT THE KETTLE
ON TO BOIL

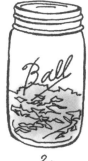

2.

FILL A QUART-SIZED
MASON JAR WITH
1 CUP OF HERB

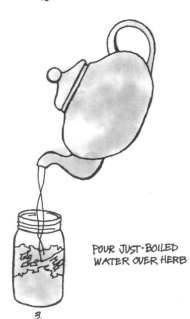

3.

POUR JUST-BOILED
WATER OVER HERB

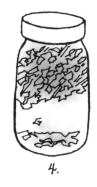

4.

STIR AND COVER.
LET SIT OVERNIGHT.

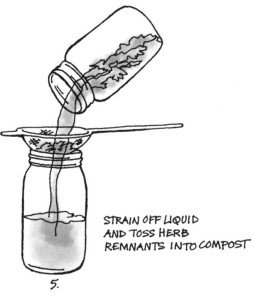

5.

STRAIN OFF LIQUID
AND TOSS HERB
REMNANTS INTO COMPOST

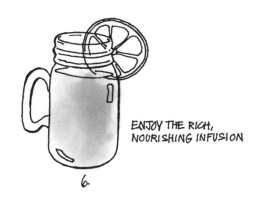

6.

ENJOY THE RICH,
NOURISHING INFUSION

I let it sit overnight while I sleep. Minerals extract slowly, and as the boiling water cools, it helps get the most nutrition out of the herbs. Although using dried herbs and boiling water ensures more complete extractions, it is still a process that takes time.

The next morning, I strain out the herbs and toss them into my compost pile. Then I enjoy sipping on the dark, nutritious liquid. You can really see and taste the minerals and nutrients that get extracted into the infusion. And as with everything, the intention you bring to this ritual of making and enjoying your infusions is important. As you are sipping, try to imagine connecting with the nutrients you are giving to all the cells of your body.

I love to have a nettles infusion in the morning because nettles can be stimulating. Often I'll have the oat straw or oat tops infusion in the evening to relax. Susun recommends you start with a single herb at a time for your infusions so you can get a feel for how your body responds.

Drinking infusions five to six times per week will ensure you are getting plenty of nutrition. Some people notice a difference right away, and for others it takes a few weeks.

less mess is best

I love making infusions, but I hate dropping little pieces of herbs on my countertops. It makes a mess, and it's a waste of good herbs! To skip the mess, use a wide-mouth canning jar and a wide-mouth canning funnel.

There are also some nifty stainless-steel strainers made to fit perfectly in quart-sized canning jars. They are usually sold for making cold-brew coffee, but they work great for herbal infusions, too.

Regardless of how you make them, when you're done, the leftover herbs make a nice mini-mulch for houseplants.

Adjusting the Flavor

Once you get a feel for how the herbs work in your body, you might want to adjust the flavor a bit. I often use one of the following natural flavor enhancers to make my infusions even more enjoyable. All these flavor enhancers have additional beneficial medicinal properties, too!

- 1 teaspoon of licorice root (adds sweetness and complexity)
- 1 teaspoon of hibiscus flowers (adds tartness)
- Pinch of stevia (adds sweetness)
- 1 teaspoon to 1 tablespoon of raw honey

Note that an infusion needs to be consumed the day you brew it. You can extend that time a day longer by storing it in the fridge, but really you should plan on drinking it right away.

The Results

The result of regular infusions is a body that's deeply nourished, full of energy, and profoundly healthy. Infusions are easy, tasty, and powerful, and when made at home, they're much more cost-effective than store-bought supplements. There's no reason not to give them a try and see how much better you can feel! Infusions are an easy addition to your daily routine and a delicious way to get dense nutrition without overloading your system.

chapter summary

- Store-bought foods no longer have the nutrition to support us.

- Vitamin and mineral supplements do not make up the difference. They may be doing more harm than good.

- High-quality supplements may give you too much of a nutrient without you knowing it.

- The best herbs for infusions are red raspberry leaf, nettles, oat straw, comfrey leaf, and red clover blossoms.

- You can customize your infusion's flavor with licorice root, hibiscus flowers, and stevia.

additional resources

For more information on infusions, check out these websites:

- www.NutritiveHerbs.com. A free series of detailed reports on the best herbs for infusions. Includes in-depth info on medicinal properties, nutritional values, historical uses, identification, how to grow, and more.

- www.HowToMakeAnInfusion.com. A free video with lots of tips and in-depth info on making infusions.

- www.HowToGrowMedicinalHerbs.com. Ramp up the potency of your herbal medicines by growing your own. This free video shows you how to grow the most popular medicinal herbs and explains when to plant, soil types, watering needs, best times to harvest, drying, and curing for the highest potency.

- www.StrongAndSexyInfusions.com. A kit with a month's supply of prepackaged herbal infusions. Includes three flavor-enhancer herbs, too.

chapter 11

growing your legacy:
seed saving,
regeneration, and more

Diane clutched the two vials as if by holding them closely she could keep her grandfather alive. We all must pass, she knew, but now that he was really gone, it hit her hard. Her husband, Kent, had asked her grandfather, Grandpa Ott, for the vials years ago. He had given them, but she and Kent had not done much with them and they were almost forgotten—until now.

Diane had such fond memories of her grandparents and especially the beautiful morning glories that covered her Grandpa Ott's porch and could be seen through the window of their home. The flowers bloomed almost the entire summer with a stunning show of gorgeous purple, with red streaks on the petals that would form a star when the flower opened in the morning.

Diane and Kent had traveled around the country on the journeys young people take. They lost some things and gained others along the way, but somehow they always managed to keep the vials with them.

Now that Grandpa Ott was gone, both Diane and Kent realized the magnitude of the responsibility they carried. In one of the two vials were the seeds from the morning glories Diane had loved so much, *Ipomoea purpurea*, and in the second vial were seeds for the German pink tomato *Solanum lycopersicum*.

The seeds had traveled from Bavaria to America with Diane's great-grandparents. The varieties had been lovingly grown, tended, and developed each year by her ancestors. What hit Diane and Kent so hard was the realization that if they did not continue to grow and collect the seeds, the lineage of that heirloom variety would die out completely.

Gone. Forever. Extinct.

Can you imagine what it must feel like to hold two small vials of seeds and realize you are the last living people to carry them forward? And if *you* don't find a way to perpetuate them, the genetics in those seeds would be permanently gone? Diane had an even bigger realization that what she was preserving was not just seeds and plants but her family's history. All heirloom seed varieties were developed by individuals over decades and centuries. None of the seeds were developed by governments or big companies. Families grew these food and medicine crops, depended on them, and refined them, season after season. These foods were as much a part of a family's story as births, weddings, and passings.

The seeds Diane and Kent carried had been held by Diane's great-grandparents on their journey from Bavaria to the United States in 1864. The morning glories growing in the summer around the farmhouse were as much a part of Diane's family history as any of life's other big moments.

Diane and Kent started to realize they were not alone. Many other people were realizing that they were "the end of the line" for an astonishing number of heirloom varieties of fruits, vegetables, flowers, herbs, and more.

In 1975, Diane placed a small ad in *Mother Earth News* magazine to reach out to other gardeners and ask if they had saved seeds they would like to share with others. The answer was a resounding yes, and the Seed Savers Exchange formally began. Hundreds of boxes of seeds began coming in the mail. Amazing varieties of beans, squashes, herbs, flowers, and more. The family stories behind the seeds came in, too. People wanted to know that their heritage would be cared for. Diane and Kent created a simple typewritten list of what was available and began regularly sending those lists to the members who wanted to continue to grow these special heirlooms.

Diane recounts this story in her memoir. The Seed Savers Exchange is still going today and has more than 13,000 members. But really, that number is paltry compared to what is needed.

More Than 90 Percent of Heirloom Varieties of Garden Crops Are Extinct, and We Are in Trouble

The USDA did a study of the number and variety of vegetables in seed catalogs available in 1903 versus those available in the National Seed Library in 1983. The results were sobering: we've lost about 93 percent of the varieties that used to exist. For example, in 1903, we had 497 varieties of lettuces, but by 1983, we were down to just 36. There used to be 544 varieties of cabbage, which have dwindled to only 28. Even the ever-popular tomato lost almost 80 percent of the heirloom genetics that used to be available. From originally 406 types, we now have 79.

"Of the more than 7,000 U.S. apple varieties that once grew in American orchards; 6,000 of them are no longer available . . . the gene pools of humanity's most basic foods are threatened," write Cary Fowler and Pat Roy Mooney in the book *Shattering: Food, Politics, and the Loss of Genetic Diversity*. In addition to the lack of backyard growers developing varieties and keeping existing strains alive, Fowler discovered that many seedbanks around the world were being destroyed or abandoned. So he took matters into his own hands. Fowler was instrumental in the creation of the Svalbard Global Seed Vault in Norway. It is a structure worthy of a James Bond movie, built hundreds of feet deep into a mountain, buried by layers and layers of ice that is supposed to never melt. It is sometimes called the "doomsday vault" because it protects the largest collection of seeds on Earth so humanity can start over in case of Armageddon-like global disasters.

While there is some solace in knowing genetics are being stored for a worst-case scenario, Svalbard is not an active seed bank in that it is not open to the public and you or I cannot access the seeds. And we don't really need sophisticated cryogenic technologies to preserve seeds effectively. The way seeds have always stayed alive is by people growing the plants, collecting the seeds, sharing them, and replanting them, year after year.

Why Does It Matter If We Don't Have as Many Varieties as We Used To?

For many years I homesteaded in Central Texas, which has a radically changeable climate. The average rainfall is 34 inches, in theory. But averages are very deceiving. We once had a 4-year drought when it rained only about 16 inches each year. The land was baked, cracked open, with almost everything dead or dying. The entire state was tinderbox dry. The drought culminated in 2011 with large parts of Texas in flames. I've never seen my farm dogs so nervous. Although they normally hated riding in the cars or trucks, they'd push their noses and then their bodies into the cab as soon as I cracked open the door to find some relief and safety. I lived in Bastrop County, near the epicenter of the Bastrop Complex fires, and it was just by the grace of God our homestead did not burn down.

And as I said, averages can be very deceiving. Sometimes we had years with more than 60 inches of rain. In 2017, Hurricane Harvey deposited 32 inches in a single weekend. The ground was so soaked that everywhere I went on the homestead, I sank almost to my calves. I didn't dare walk into the garden to the drowning plants because I would have destroyed the soil structure. And for the chickens, I laid out big sheets of 4×8-foot plywood as life rafts my dripping birds could stand on.

The temperature in Central Texas is also highly changeable. Some years the winters were pleasantly mild, and we ran around in T-shirts. Other years, it got down to the single digits with long icicles hanging off of the eaves.

To produce food in that radically unpredictable environment, you have to have a large diversity of different species. The most successful strategy is to plant a big selection, including everything from plants known to be drought-tolerant to those that like to be wet, some that withstand cold, and others that like the heat. You know full well you are going to lose some, some will struggle, and some will thrive.

The main point is, having a diversity of cultivars of crops is essential. And now more than ever, crop diversity is essential for human survival. Many of the varieties of heirlooms we've lost had properties of tolerance or production that would be immensely useful right now, especially as our climate changes.

Homestead Livestock Is Also in Danger

The family cow used to be a significant part of a family's wealth. In fact, many of our financial concepts and terms are derived from livestock ownership. A "cash cow" refers to a cow that provides good milk with little work. The milk is a steady stream of income equivalent to interest or dividends. "Capital gains" comes from the calf the cow produces each year. "All hat and no cows" describes someone who is bluffing about their supposed (but nonexistent) wealth. And "Don't put all your eggs in one basket" refers to the wisdom of diversity in investments.

In early American history, a common family cow was the milking Devon. Devon cattle are a sturdy, good-natured breed that is able to thrive under rugged conditions. The Devons had tasty beef and also gave good quantities of high-fat milk. Remember that throughout history (and contrary to our momentary modern whim), fat was considered a very good thing. The best cheeses come from milk with a high fat content. And if you like cream in your coffee, you should try the real stuff sometime. The Devon oxen were also known to be quick and good pullers. They were the draft animals of choice on the Oregon Trail. Devons could be seen everywhere on small farms and homesteads dotted across the landscape of our young country.

As the celebration of the two hundredth year of America's existence drew near in 1976, several living history museums such as Old Sturbridge Village in Sturbridge, Massachusetts, and Plimoth Plantation in Plymouth, Massachusetts, wanted to upgrade the accuracy of their representations of early American life. From the historical records, the Devon cattle stood out as the most common animal in use and a centerpiece of American homesteads. But the museums ran into a big problem. There were almost no Devon cattle in existence anymore.

The difficulty they had in finding this once-popular breed was the inspiration for the founding of the organization now known as the Livestock Conservancy. Like the Seed Savers Exchange, the Livestock Conservancy and a host of smaller, breed-specific organizations have been doing as much as they can to keep these valuable livestock genetics alive.

In the decades since we have moved away from backyard food production, homesteading, and small farms, the animals we once relied upon have slowly disappeared, too. It's very simple—if we don't tend them and use them, they die off. Have you ever seen a red wattle hog? A Belgian hare? A Meishan pig? Or a miniature Dexter cow? The idea that livestock could go extinct isn't something many of us have ever worried about. But it's a serious problem. So many useful and productive breeds are on the verge of disappearing. Like the genetics of plant crops, many are already completely gone. Those breeds were the results of painstaking work of individuals and families over years, decades, and even centuries of careful selection.

I spoke with Jeanette Beranger, senior program manager for the Livestock Conservancy, to discuss the importance of the heritage breeds and the critical role they play in true food resiliency. Most people don't realize that the animals being used in large-scale commercial agriculture have been so specially bred for eating industrially produced grain that the animals are not viable in what should be their natural environment. For example, commercial breeds of cattle cannot fatten up on pasture grass, and many would die if they were to only graze on the grasses their ancestors thrived on.

The Cornish rock cross chicken, which is the darling of commercial meat production, is specifically developed to put on weight with incredible speed. And they don't stop growing. If not processed within a very short time of maturity, they will gain so much more weight that they will die because they can no longer walk.

Many of the animals used in commercial meat factories cannot breed naturally on their own.

In contrast, the traditional, historic breeds contain essential attributes for survival and self-sufficiency—fertility, foraging ability, good temperaments, longevity, maternal instincts, ability to mate naturally, and resistance to diseases and parasites. Ensuring these heritage genetics stay vibrant is imperative for our survival.

I asked Jeanette what advice she would give to anyone who wanted to become a protector of a heritage breed. Here is what she recommended:

> Don't take on a breed just because it's cute—take it on because it has practical uses in your region (such as enjoying cold weather, producing something you need, or the ability to forage on what grows in your area). For genetic resiliency, encourage others in your area to also become

champions for the same breed. A group of backyard producers can have enough genetic diversity even though each family only has a few animals. Start out with less-than-perfect representatives of the breed—perhaps some of the "culls." They are less expensive, and you have a lot to learn in the beginning. As your animal husbandry skills improve, you can take on, and continue to develop, the best of the breed.

Why We Should *Not* Pursue Sustainability

I have Finian Makepeace to thank for helping me understand why sustainability is really not a good goal. Finian works with Kiss the Ground, a soil advocacy group. Finian and his cohorts realize that soil destruction is at the root of all real food production problems, both for plant and animal species. When he once told me bluntly that sustainable was "stupid," I was shocked. I'd thought Finian and I had a lot in common. We are both all about soil, and understanding it is a key part of any solutions to the food supply problems going forward. We are both active advocates of soil microbiology.

But his reasoning makes sense. As he points out, sustainability means "to sustain"—to keep things where they are, to maintain the current state, to hold the status quo. And that is not acceptable. The planet has already endured so much destruction, we need to do much better than just maintain the current levels—we have to work on regeneration.

Finian is absolutely correct, and I've been careful about using the word "sustainability" ever since. We have to focus on regeneration. There are many organizations with "sustainable development goals," and that is a great start. I get that their intent is sincere, but language matters, and I'd like to see those organizations upgrade their focus to "regenerative development goals."

The Biggest Myth of a Resilient Local Food Supply

I have never met anyone who didn't want to have a more resilient local food supply. Citizens, city councils, state governments, and world leaders are all urging for better, healthier food available locally. But there is a huge misunderstanding of exactly what it takes to achieve that.

Most people assume it means we need to encourage a lot more local organic farms and farmers to produce the food. Many proposals have been put forward with the idea of a city or town surrounded by hundreds or thousands of smaller organic farms, ranches, orchards, and other productive farm enterprises. Some have called this a community foodshed, similar to the concept of a community watershed.

Actually, the model of a city surrounded on its outskirts by a patchwork of food production is historically a very successful system. F. H. King's *Farmers of Forty Centuries*, originally published in 1911, describes in detail how extremely dense populations in Japan, China, and Korea were supported by networks of small farms producing massive amounts of food, century after century, without depleting their soils.

We absolutely do need to rebuild the small farm network that once supported much of the American population not all that long ago. But there is one hugely important factor almost everyone neglects when they talk about resilient local food systems—we also need to have an army of backyard food producers.

Backyard gardens are more stable economically. The savings in fuel is obvious—essentially no transport, packaging, or processing happens when you step from your backyard into the kitchen. Backyard producers tend to also be much more waterwise and use up to 80 percent less water than commercial farmers. And there is significantly less food wasted, the loads on landfills are reduced, and there is greater conservation and cycling of nutrients. Believe me, when you are growing your own, you don't throw it out.

But the biggest reason you cannot have a resilient local food supply without an army of backyard producers is genetics. As just discussed, it is imperative that we work today to preserve the heritage species we have and to develop more. Most farmers, regardless of the size of their operation, do not have the time to experiment, test, and trial new varieties of plants and animals. Farmers have more than enough work to do to produce what they can to earn a living. They simply don't have time to try out a lot of new things.

Backyard producers, on the other hand, do have the time. Even though our space is much more limited, we have the luxury of being able to experiment. Local backyard producers help their local farmers by testing out varieties, experimenting, and refining processes. Large companies, governmental stations, and university researchers are focused exclusively on chemical agriculture and the needs of megascale agribusiness. They have entirely different motives and requirements for production. They do not produce heirloom varieties of plants. They do not produce genetics useful for small-scale production.

All our heritage genetics come from backyard gardens or small homesteads. They have all come from people like your great-grandparents, who developed useful varieties without microscopes, DNA sequencers, electricity, or the internet. It is highly unlikely they had degrees in biology or genetics. Yet they produced all the wonderful tastes, resilience, and practicality of the heirloom genetics we have left. It is just astonishing what people with very humble means can do.

My friend Leslie is bringing this tradition back. Leslie has a small garden of less than 100 square feet, and she works three part-time jobs to make ends meet. Leslie's garden had a big problem—it was a magnet for the dreaded squash vine borer. None of her squash plants ever survived the ravages of these insects. But instead of reaching for chemicals or complaining, Leslie decided to turn this problem into an opportunity and a gift for everyone in her region.

Leslie is keenly aware of how important squash is as a staple crop—and it will become even more important as the global food crisis escalates. There are lots of wonderful recipes to turn it into all kinds of dishes, and the winter squashes can be stored for many months in areas where it's too cold and you need to depend on food storage to get through a winter. It grows so prolifically, and it is a very important source of nutrition and calories.

Leslie started experimenting with different varieties of squashes that were resistant to the vine borers. Scouring old texts, chasing rumors, digging through seed catalogs, and trying many different types, she stumbled across one variety of a little pumpkin squash known as tatume (*Cucurbita pepo*) that not only survived but actually thrived in her yard. Impressed but still not fully convinced she'd solved her problem for good, Leslie continued to grow the tatume squashes in her garden and watch the results closely. Then, at the beginning of the next growing season, she gave out tatume starts to as many friends as would take them. They all grew them in an experiment to see how the plants would thrive in different locations. At the end of several growing seasons, Leslie and a ragtag group of about a dozen backyard producers definitively concluded that yes, the tatume was a variety that could outwit the vine borer.

There are so many other stories like this about backyard champions. David the Good, also known as "The Survival Gardener," is the author of many great gardening books. David was playing around with different tatume squashes by running a big landrace project in his yard, which meant he was collecting seeds of different cultivars of the same varieties, planting them all together, and letting them crossbreed. He'd then select the seeds from the most vigorous and tasty squashes that were produced. You can buy the same-named cultivar from different seed houses and end up with varying results. Although the seeds are technically from the same cultivar, because they've been grown and collected in different places, they often have slightly different characteristics. Growing them all together and letting them crossbreed is a way to add genetic diversity and strength back into a particular line.

David had gotten some great results from his landrace, and he offered to send me some seeds from his winners to try out. I was thrilled when his envelope arrived with its precious cargo. And then my inner prankster just couldn't help herself. It was autumn, and I had also been growing a version of these cute little pumpkin squashes. I harvested a particularly beautiful specimen, wrapped it carefully, and shipped the full-grown squash back to David. I included this note in the box:

Hey David. Wow, you were so right! These seeds are amazing. I planted them last week, and look how quickly it grew. You are really onto something here.

David and I couldn't stop laughing when I got the phone call from him.

Discover and Create Your Legacy

When Cary Fowler spoke to audiences about the loss of heirloom species and the need for their protection, he would take out a list of the 6,000 varieties of apples that no longer exist. He didn't tell the group these were extinct apple varieties, but simply asked everyone to look them over and see if they could find a family name in the list.

Perhaps they could recognize the surname of an uncle or their mother's maiden name.

Cary said that, invariably, with every audience, about two-thirds of the room recognized a family name in the list. Then he told them the name was an apple variety developed by one of their ancestors, but the trees are now gone. Cary himself found a "fowler apple," which had been developed by an ancestor of his. He jokingly tells everyone that it is described as "a beautiful fruit with an unruly growth habit." Who knows what other very desirable characteristics the fowler apple may have had, such as resistance to blight, or a wide range of chill hours, or something else that could be immensely useful.

If you live in Texas, you'll want to be sure you know about the "Pop's Porter" tomato. Developed by Kenneth Glowka, who is affectionately known as "Pops" by his 4 sons, 11 grandchildren, and hundreds of friends and neighbors, the "Pop's Porter" is the name of a small to mid-sized tomato that miraculously is able to grow in the stifling Texas summer heat. Kenneth will be the first to tell you it isn't the tastiest thing ever, but to have some kind of fresh tomato to enjoy in the summer is a delight. And his kids continue to grow it. If you live in Texas, you will certainly want to grow other, tastier varieties in the autumn and spring, but what he achieved is really an accomplishment. My neighbors and I all think of Pops and tell stories about him while we're eating fried okra and tomatoes in August.

You'd get to name any new cultivars you develop, too! And you can certainly name your farm, even if it's just a backyard. What better gift to give your family, your community, and all the lives who come after you than the gift of food? What better way to be remembered?

Using Competition for Good

A few years ago, I purchased a small farmhouse in Colorado. Whenever I buy a property, it is always for the yard—the house is a secondary consideration. As the seller showed me around the grounds, he proudly patted the trunk of an ancient cherry tree and announced the variety had won the World's Fair in 1934 for the best cherries. Based on the huge girth of the old trees in the yard, those very trees were probably planted in that timeframe, if not earlier. By the way, those trees are still producing delicious cherries today as I write this, although I know I'll need to be starting some new younger ones soon.

Regional fairs and their friendly competitions have historically been a great way for people to showcase their backyard accomplishments. They were also how growers exchanged and shared information. Local farmers could learn about new varieties and techniques, and the fairs helped strengthen the entire region. Some of this exists today and can still be very powerful. When my children were very young, they won blue ribbons at the plant show sponsored by the local organic gardening club. Those ribbons are still treasured memorabilia from their childhoods. If we make these events part of our culture again, we can unleash a lot of talent.

Years ago, I visited Cuba to interview survivors of its "special period," the economic collapse after the Soviet Union broke apart and the Cuban economy, which was largely propped up by exporting sugar at inflated prices to the USSR, collapsed. The Cuban economy quickly tanked by 60 percent, the lights went out, and the water stopped running. During this period, the average Cuban lost 20 pounds due to food scarcity. Overnight, the social structure turned completely upside down. The once-lowly gardeners now moved up in social status to exceed their former employers, the lawyers and doctors.

It is clear that our global economy is shifting away from a consumptive model toward that of small-scale production. It will definitely be a difficult transition, but we do not have to go through the severity of the Cuban experience. We can use regional events to resurrect the local food movement and to offer status, honor, and recognition for those who are helping rebuild the local foodsheds. And we can do it before it becomes a sheer necessity.

I regularly do podcasts with CEOs of successful startups and executives of large organizations. These are people who have mostly bootstrapped their way up, and they are managing budgets in the tens and hundreds of millions of dollars with teams from a few dozen to thousands of employees. The reason I interview them is because they also grow their own food. These men and women are incredibly talented and driven. They could afford to buy whatever they wanted, of course, so they are not growing food to save money. You can listen to the podcasts, but I'll give you the punchline: every one of them says the primary reason they spend half an hour to an hour per day in their backyards working with the earth is for stress relief.

But what really has astonished me is how proud they are of what they've grown. Prior to our interviews, these super-busy professionals will literally send me an unsolicited album full of photos of big tables laden with recently harvested homegrown tomatoes, or images of cartons of multicolored eggs, snapshots of their pantries full of homemade pickles, or glamour shots of their beautiful hens. They have nowhere else to show them off. Similarly, when I go to events to speak, invariably people come up and show me photos on their phones of their gardens, orchards, and rabbits. They are so excited about what they've created, and they want to share. There should be outlets to encourage that.

If you are the kind of person gifted with the knack of organizing events, consider this a personal call from me to you to create or resurrect a regional harvest festival. And fortunately, you won't have to completely reinvent the wheel because we still have many resources we can reinvigorate.

4-H and Future Farmers of America (FFA) are open to adult participation, and both organizations welcome and need volunteers. Both have excellent programs for animal husbandry, growing and processing food, and other homesteading skills. The Grange organization, which was founded after the Civil War, is still in existence in many areas and looking for new members.

Master Gardener programs are also great resources for in-depth learning about how to grow food, and they organize great events around celebrating production. Many have a commercial agriculture orientation, but more and more are switching to organic and regenerative offerings. The networking is fabulous, and the potlucks are amazing.

Growing Supernatural

In Chapter 2, I introduced the idea that there are some extraordinary exceptions to conventional gardening wisdom. If you recall, most plants have a preferred temperature zone where they like to grow. Warm season plants die when there is a freeze. Cold season plants bolt (or go to seed), or burn up and die, in the heat. And

99.99 percent of the time this is true. But there are incredible stories of some outliers that have done extraordinary things.

For example, basil is an herb that just loves, loves, loves the heat. It does not do well in cold weather, and it certainly dies in a freeze. But Stephanie Syson, a talented and dedicated biodynamic farmer who grows medicinal herbs, had an amazing experience growing basil. Stephanie grows for the sheer love of it and for the joy it brings her, and the medicinal herbs she produces are extraordinary. Stephanie loves to grow holy basil, and one season she gave a stronger blessing than usual to her seeds and then grew them with her usual loving care. At the end of the season, she didn't get around to composting or turning under the basil plant remnants as she normally would. One morning after an arctic blast came through the valley, Stephanie was astonished to see her basil plants happily peeking up and growing through the snow.

I experienced something similar years before I ever thought about growing food. I was an ex-pat living and working in Hong Kong. Flats (a.k.a. apartments) in Hong Kong are notoriously long, narrow, and dark with small windows at only one end and essentially no sunlight. My good friend Deborah Chan was a reiki master who regularly held classes in the living room of her modest Causeway Bay flat. Reiki is a form of energy healing, and Deborah taught groups of people how to focus their innate healing energy for themselves or for others. What was astonishing was that Deborah had a couple of small pots of flowers that never got sunlight but continually bloomed. I didn't know enough about plants at that time to know the species, and to be honest, I'm not much into ornamentals anyway—I prefer to focus on food-producing plants. But many of Deborah's students were knowledgeable, and one was a botanist. The plants in Deborah's living room normally required a lot of sunlight to produce flowers, but there was no sunlight, ever, in her living room, just a few incandescent lamps on the end tables by the couch. We were all mystified by the beautiful blooms that were growing impossibly. The only thing we could attribute it to was the intense healing energy that was regularly generated in the room.

There has been a scattering of scientific studies on the topic of the power of intention to influence plant growth. I am absolutely fascinated by this and the potential for better crop production, especially for medicinal herbs. Many gardeners have done DIY experiments of this kind with fascinating results, and my community at

The Grow Network is interested and willing to help look at this new frontier. I am looking for independent researchers who are interested in the project. If that is you, please reach out. There is so much more to explore and understand, and we have a lot of work to do. Maybe one day we can quantify these effects and even show an improved nutritional or medicinal quality based on our focused attention. If you want to keep up to date on whatever experiments I've managed to get going, sign up at www.BlessingsCloud.com. I believe this is the new frontier for food and medicine.

chapter summary

- Most people are not aware of the importance of plant and animal genetics and how much we've lost in the last decades.

- Sustainability is not good enough—we must focus on regeneration.

- Regional competitions and fairs are a great way to honor innovative backyard producers and experimenters.

- You can create a truly useful legacy in your backyard.

additional resources

For more information, check out these websites:
- www.BlessingsCloud.com. Sign up here if you want to keep up to date and/ or participate in experiments and research in using the power of thought and intention.

- www.MyPlaceOnEarth.com is a short quiz that helps you determine the bioregion you live in and connects you up with resources and other people who are in regions that grow similar plants and animals.

A Final Farewell

Well, my friend, we have come to the end of the book. It's been quite a journey. I hope I've shown you that there is much more to wealth than simply money. Health and happiness can't be bought, but they can be grown in a backyard. Good food, good friends, good memories—this is what makes you rich.

You've seen that it is fairly easy to grow half of your own food. All you really need is a 100-square-foot garden, six laying hens, and a small home rabbitry. And in growing half, your life will change dramatically for the better. The *process* of growing food is more health-enhancing than eating the nutritious products, although that is nice, too. The stress relief, gentle exercise, sunshine, distance from electronics, and fresh air are magical elixirs. You've seen that production is much, much more than counting calories—it's extending your immediate community far beyond your circle of humans to include many other species of plants and animals. I believe interspecies relations are the frontier for agriculture.

You've opened to the possibility that there may be much more healthy food already growing right now in your front yard or your local park or greenbelt. That you might have a very important role in helping restore wilderness. And those weeds you've been fighting and trying to kill, if you make peace with them, you might actually find they are great medicine and nutrition.

You've learned how simple and easy it is to make medicines at home, and you've gotten a taste of the potential power they contain. And you've come to realize how important you are in revitalizing our pool of food genetics and helping regenerate the earth. I hope to see you, grinning from ear to ear, holding that blue ribbon for the tastiest strawberry or the healthiest rabbit. And I hope you realize that the very best way to be remembered by your great-great-grandchildren is by leaving them a journal of herbal medicines, or the plants or animals you helped caretake.

It's not often that a writer gets to pen a book that solves global problems. And I am not claiming to have figured out everything. But it continues to astonish me how such a simple and humble act of growing and sharing food, making medicine, and loving one another is the solution to so many of our modern concerns.

Please.

grow

Acknowledgments

This book could have never come about without the years of support from the entire Grow Network—our members, moderators, admins, volunteers, and team. Ruth Reyes, Linzi Searcy, Merin Porter, Jimerson Adkins, Nikki Follis, Mary Korman, and Anthony Tamayo: you have been pulling with me for a long time. Thank you.

To my kids, Ryan and Kimber, I am so grateful you've shown me the truth that the children are the mother of the woman. Thanks to Dave and the entire Glowka clan, with whom we've shared so many good times. And to my family, who has supported me for as long as I've been on this planet: Frank, Anna, Shelly, George, Ronnie, Todd, Mary-Anne, Selene, Guy, and Linda.

This book could not have come about without the help from Anna Petkovich and Celeste Fine of Park and Fine Literary; the awesome drawings from Alexis Seabrook; and all the behind-the-scenes work of Lucia Watson and her team at Avery. Thank you.

Index

index   271

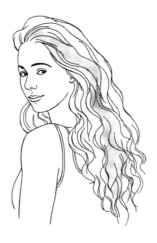

About the Author

....

Marjory Wildcraft is the founder of The Grow Network, which is a movement of people who are stopping the destruction of Earth via homegrown food. Marjory's work focuses on building deep community resilience, restoring heirloom genetics in gardens and livestock, and advancing the return to natural medicine. Marjory hosts the annual Home Grown Food and Home Medicine Summits, which reach hundreds of thousands of viewers every year.

Beloved for her humorous, nonjudgmental, get -'er-done style, Marjory raised two teenagers in Central Texas and currently is working with local organic farming communities in Rincón, Puerto Rico, and Paonia, Colorado. When she's not building an online network, being "Mom," and tending her family's food supply, Marjory loves playing, running, doing gymnastics, ka-rate, acquiring skills from the Paleolithic era (yes, she is part cavewoman!), and experimenting with anything and everything.

You can reach Marjory directly by going to the Grow Network forums, where she posts and interacts with her community on her latest adventures.